FAMILY MEDICINE

Published by:
Lotus Press

A GUIDE TO FAMILY MEDICINE

Dr. Rajeev Sharma

M.D., D.Lit.

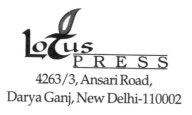

4263/3, Ansari Road,
Darya Ganj, New Delhi-110002

Lotus Press
4263/3, Ansari Road, Darya Ganj, New Delhi-110002.
Ph.: 32903912, 23280047, 9811594448
E-mail: lotus_press@sify.com ❑ www.lotuspress.co.in

A Guide to Family Medicine
© 2008, Lotus Press
ISBN: 81-8382-162-6

Attentions Readers:
Every effort is made to ensure accuracy of material, but the publisher, printer and author will not be held responsible for any inadvertent error (s). In case of any dispute, all legal matters to be settled under Delhi Jurisdiction only.

Published by: Lotus Press, New Delhi.
Printed by: Anand Sons, Delhi.
Laser Typeset by: Aruna Enterprises, Delhi-110 094

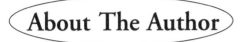

About The Author

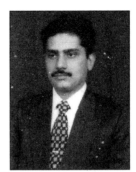

Dr. Rajeev Sharma

Dr. Rajeev Sharma is an eminent consultant of Homoeo-pathy, Yoga, Naturopathy and Alternative Medicine in India. He has written more than two hundred twenty five books (225) in Hindi and English and around one thousand articles which have been published in various newspapers and magazines. He is also an Editorial Board Member of the prestigious Asian Homoeopathic Journal besides many other newspapers and magazines.

Dr. Rajeev Sharma has written books on ayurveda, homoeo-pathy, yoga, naturopathy, accupressure, magnetotherapy, water-therapy, massage and aromatherapy etc., and on all major ailments.

Dr. Rajeev Sharma is Medical Advisor to Ralson Remedies (a homoeopathic manufacturer), and Dixit Pharmacy (Ayurvedic Manufacturer), Sr. Medical Officer U.P. Govt. He has received several prizes for his outstanding achievements. He has been awarded the *Best Author Prize in Hindi* by the Ministry of Health and Family Welfare, Government of India and *Sarjana Puraskar* by *U.P. Hindi Sansthan*, Lucknow. He has delivered talks on All India Radio and Total T.V. and lectures on Alternative Medicine in various Government and Non-government Organisations. He has written Advt. Scripts for the products of several companies.

He has established an institute through which you can get certificates by correspondence in Accupressure, Massage, Yoga, Water Therapy, Diet Therapy, Naturopathy, Colour Therapy and Reiki besides other paramedical courses.

He is providing literature on Personality Development and Life-Style Management.

Dr. Rajeev Sharma is also a social activist. He has worked a lot against Addiction and Prevention of AIDS. He has worked for population and pollution control and human rights and has received the World Human Rights Promotion Award. His name has been published in *LIMCA BOOK OF RECORDS,* 2005. He has developed a website too :- www.newkamasutra.com

Dr. Rajeev Sharma is National President of an NGO UTKRISHTA BHARAT (An All India Association of Socio-Cultural Religious and Sports Activities).

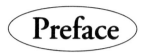

Preface

Normally, a family consists of husband-wife, two kids and grand parents. This book "A Guide to Family Medicine" contains all the information from head to toe which provide complete information including symptoms/treatment/complications/ selfcare and appropriate homoeopathic and ayurvedic medicines. So, this is a useful book for younger as well as elders.

This book provides simple treatment plans for conjunctivitis, epistaxis, sore throat, toothache, common cold, cough, diarrhoea, constipation, gas, haemorrhoids, bladder infection, joint pain, back pain, skin infections, grief, insomnia, headache, impotency, dysmenrrohea, fever, hypertension etc.

Hope readers will find it useful.

Dr. Rajeev Sharma

Srijan—Aarogya Jyoti®
Palm—11/03, Shipra Sun City
Ghaziabad (U.P.)
Ph.: 0120-6460127
email: sharmarajeev108@rediffmail.com

Contents

Eye-Ear-Nose-Throat Disorders

Care should be taken for Eyes, Ears, Nose, Throat in all Seasons. We should avoid movement in dust and taken precaution in winters and summers. We should not eat much sour spicy food.

EYE DISORDERS

Conjunctivitis

Conjunctivitis, also known as pinkeye, is an acute inflammation of the conjunctiva of the eye, which is a thin protective lining of the eyelids and eyeball. It is caused by bacterial or viral infection or an allergic sensitivity to an irritant.

Symptoms

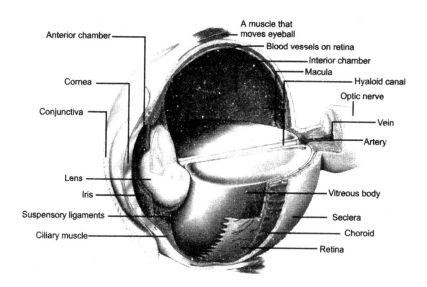

The eye appears red and bloodshot, and there is often lots of watering and a clear or purulent (pus) discharge, depending on whether the infection is viral or bacterial. The eyelids are usually swollen, intense itching occurs with allergic conjunctivitis. The eye feels irritated and painful, and there is a burning sensation or a feeling that something is in the eye.

Complications

Conjunctivitis may become chronic or may damage the eye if left untreated.

Homoeopathic Medicines

- ☞ If the main symptom is puffy swelling of the eyelids, give Apis.
- ☞ For conjunctivitis in newborns, think of Argentum nitricum.
- ☞ When fever, redness, and throbbing pain are prominent, Belladonna is the medicine.
- ☞ If the main symptom is excessive, irritating tears, give Euphrasia.
- ☞ If the discharge is thick, creamy, and yellow green in a whiny, moody person, give Pulsatilla.
- ☞ If burning in the eyes is prominent in a lazy, philosophical egoist, give Sulphur.

Self Care and Home Remedies

- ☞ Apply a clean washcloth that has been dipped in cold water and wrung out over the eyes. Replace it when it gets warm.
- ☞ Rub the hands together vigorously and place over the closed eyes for one minute.
- ☞ Do not touch the other eye after you have touched the infected eye, to avoid spreading the infection.

☞ Use sterile Euphrasia eyedrops to soothe the eyes, a few drops in each eye after you have touched the infected eye, to avoid spreading the infection.

☞ Use sterile Euphrasia eyedrops to soothe the eyes, a few drops in each eye several times a day.

☞ Dissolve one fourth teaspoon of salt in one cup of water.

☞ Use three cotton balls soaked in the water to swipe the edge of the eyelids from inside to outside. Discard after using once. Repeat four times a day.

☞ Take beta carotene (50,000 IU per day) or Vitamin A (25,000 IU per day). Take Vitamin C (500 mg, two times per day).

STYE

A stye is an infection of a sweat or oil gland in the eyelid.

Symptoms

The first symptoms are usually pain, redness, swelling, and tenderness of the edge of the eyelid, followed by the appearance of a small, round, tender, hardened area. Tears, sensitivity to light, and a feeling of a foreign body in the eye may follow.

Complications

Complications are rare, but styes are often recurrent.

Homoeopathic Medicines

☞ If the styes are pus filled and sensitive to drafts, give Hepar sulphuris.

☞ For styes of the right eye with lots of dryness, look at Lycopodium.

☞ If the main symptom is profuse, thick, yellowish discharge from the eye, give Pulsatilla.

☞ For dry, painful eyes in a woman who never gets angry, give Staphysagria.

☞ If the edges of the lids are red, burning, itchy, and irritated, give Sulphur.

Self Care and Home Remedies
☞ Keep the eye clean.
☞ Place compresses soaked in hot water on the eyelid for ten minutes several times a day to bring the stye to a head and allow it to drain.
☞ Give Vitamin C (500 mg two times a day) for immune support.

EAR DISORDERS

Ear Infection
Ear infections may be either internal or external. Otitis media, a middle ear infection, occurs behind the eardrum. Otitis externa, an outer ear infection, occurs in the ear canal outside the drum. Acute middle ear infections are associated with bacteria. Chronic middle ear inflammation may come from chronic bacterial infection or a buildup of fluid, usually caused by allergic reactions. Infants who are exposed to solid food and cow's milk too early may develop significant food allergies which are directly correlated with chronic ear infections. The allergies often begin right after the child is weaned from breast feeding.

Symptoms
Middle ear infections cause acute pain, a clogged or blocked sensation in the ear with some temporary loss of hearing, and bulging of the eardrum. More rarely, the eardrum can rupture, discharging pus and fluid into the ear canal. Chronic ear infections cause redness of the eardrum and pressure and blockage in the ears with some, usually reversible, hearing loss.

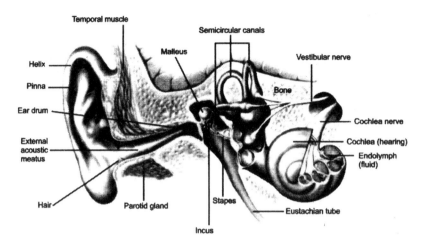

Complications

Following a rupture, the eardrum will usually repair itself, but may leave scarring. Chronic ear infections may cause hearing loss, which usually resolves when the fluid drains or disappears. In chronic middle ear inflammation with an allergic basis ("glue ear") antibiotics are ineffective on a long-term basis, and the causative allergic responses must be addressed. Even in acute ear infections, antibiotics may not shorten the course of illness. Conventional physicians often recommend surgical insertion of tubes into the eardrums to drain off the fluid, in order to prevent chronic hearing loss which may interfere with language development in young children.

Homeopathic Medicines

☞ If a child quickly develops an ear infection after playing in the cold air, she needs Aconite.

☞ If the child has intense, throbbing pain in the right ear, a bright red face, and a fever of 103°F or higher, give Belladonna.

☞ For fussy children whose ear infections are associated with teething Chamomilla is best.

☞ Children who scream with pain during an ear infection may need Hepar sulphuris, Belladonna, or Chamomilla.

☞ If mercurius is needed, there is likely to be bad breath, a coated tongue, excessive saliva, and bad smelling perspiration.

☞ Mild, moody children who cry easily and want to be held and caressed during an ear infection are likely to need Pulsatila.

☞ If Silica is needed, there wil generally be a tendency to swollen glands, excessive bad smelling perspiration, and possibly a history of dental problems.

Self Care and Home Remedies

☞ Mullein garlic oil drops, three drops in the affected ear three times daily. Warm the oil bottle under the faucet first. Put a piece of cotton in the ear after inserting drops to prevent the oil from coming out. If there is a tendency for the infection to spread from one ear to the other, put the drops in both ears.

☞ Alternating hot and cold compresses to the affected ear.

☞ Beta-carotene: 50,000 units daily in acute cases; 25,000 units daily in chronic cases.

☞ It is often helpful to remove milk products from the diet, at least temporarily.

☞ Goat's milk is a good substitute for cow's milk.

THROAT DISORDERS

Mumps

Mumps is a contagious viral infection of the parotid gland in the upper jaw, just below and in front of the ears and other salivary glands. Mumps usually occurs in children, but can be more serious in adults.

Symptoms

The primary symptoms are moderate to high fever with chills, and painful swelling of the parotid glands and other salivary glands with fatigue and loss of appetite.

Complications

In men past puberty, the main complication of mumps is painful inflammation of the testes which can, in rare cases, cause sterility. Meningoencephalitis, which resembles bacterial meningitis, is characterised by a headache, stiff neck, and, rarely, convulsions or a coma. Pancreatitis with nausea, vomiting, and pain in the abdomen sometimes occurs at the end of the first week of mumps, and gets completely better in about a week.

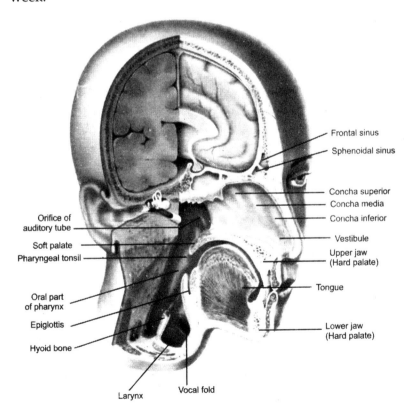

Frontal sinus

Sphenoidal sinus

Concha superior
Concha media
Concha inferior

Orifice of
auditory tube

Vestibule

Soft palate
Pharyngeal tonsil

Upper jaw
(Hard palate)

Oral part
of pharynx

Tongue

Epiglottis

Lower jaw
(Hard palate)

Hyoid bone

Larynx   Vocal fold

Homoeopathic Medicines

- ☞ Mercurius is the most common medicine used for mumps.
- ☞ Phytolacca is used to treat stony hard parotid glands with pain extending to on swallowing.
- ☞ Carbo vegetabils is used for mumps when exhaustion and bloating are prominent symptoms.
- ☞ Pulsatilla and Carbo vegetabilis are both used when mumps causes inflammation of the testes or breasts.
- ☞ Pulsatilla is appropriate when the child or adult is weepy and clingy with a lot of swelling in the testes or breasts.
- ☞ Less common medicines which help inflammation of the testes during or after mumps are Abrotanum and Jaborandi.
- ☞ Abrotannum is used to treat a large swollen parotid gland that goes down as the testes become swollen. It is given to irritable, cruel children with a failure to thrive.
- ☞ Jaborandi treats mumps with increased sweating and salivation, and parotid glands double their usual size. This medicine has been used to shorten the duration of the disease.

Self Care and Home Remedies

Rest

- ☞ Eat soft foods to reduce the need for chewing.
- ☞ Avoid spicy and sour foods and drinks, such as citrus fruit and other juices, which may cause pain by stimulating the salivary glands.
- ☞ Isolate the person with mumps to avoid spreading the infection to those who have not had it.
- ☞ Take Vitamin C, 500 mg two times daily for children four years or older.

- Use a carrot poultice to relieve swelling. Blend two to three carrots, place in a cloth or cheesecloth and apply under chin for two to eight hours.

Sore Throats

Pharyngitis is an inflammation of the pharynx or throat which is usually associated with a virus or, as in the case of a strep throat, a bacteria.

Symptoms

The most distressing symptom is usually a mild to severe pain in the throat, which may extend to the ears. There may be a simultaneous upperrespiratory infection, bronchitis, or flu.

Complications

An untreated Group A Beta-hemolytic strep infection may lead to rheumatic fever or joint problems.

Homoeopathic Medicines

- ☞ For throat pain of very rapid onset with a high fever, give Aconite or Belladonna.
- ☞ If it feels better from cold drinks, first look at Apis.
- ☞ If the main symptom is swelling, give Apis or Phytolacca.
- ☞ For very red sore throats, the best medicines are Belladonna and Apis.
- ☞ For a burning, right sided sore throat in a person with a bright red face and ear pain, give Belladonna.
- ☞ For right sided sore throats, think of Belladonna, Apis, Lycopodium, Phytolacca, and Mercurius iodatus flavus.
- ☞ The medicines to give for sore throats that have the most pain on swallowing are Lachesis, Hepar sulphuris, Belladonna, and Mercurius.
- ☞ For left sided sore throats, consider Lachesis first, then, more rarely, Mercurius iodatus ruber.

☞ The first medicine to consider for sore throats that start on the left then move to the right is Lachesis.

☞ For sore throats that begin on the right then go to the left, look at Lycopodium.

☞ If the sore throat feels better from warm drinks, think first of Lycopodium.

Self Care and Home Remedies

☞ Gargle with warm salt water three times a day.

☞ Gargle with one teaspoon of Calendula tincture in one cup of warm water.

☞ Suck on zinc lozenges. (Avoid any lozenges with menthol, camphor, or eucalyptus, since they interfere with homoeopathic treatment.)

☞ Take Vitamin C (3000 mg a day) in divided doses of 500 mg. Cut the dose in half for a child and give a maximum of 250 mg to a baby.

☞ Take echinacea and goldenseal tincture in water (one half teaspoon every two hours, up to six doses a day).

☞ Avoid dairy products and sweets.

☞ Drink one to two glasses of fresh carrot juice per day.

NOSE DISORDERS

Epistaxis

Nose-bleeds are simply spontaneous bleeding from the nose. They are caused by infections of the nose and sinuses, dryness and cracking of the nasal mucous membranes, ruptured blood vessels and trauma. Vigorous nose blowing or nose picking can sometimes induce a nosebleed. More serious chronic conditions, such as high blood pressure, arteriosclerosis, and bleeding diseases like hemophilia, may be involved.

Symptoms

Blood or blood tinged mucus either drips or is blown from the nose. Clots may form in the nose. Be careful if you remove these clots, or the nose may begin bleeding again.

Complications

Low blood volume and anemia may occur if the nosebleed will not stop and blood loss is extreme. If a nosebleed will not stop readily with direct pressure and homoeopathic medicines, seek medical attention to find the source of the nosebleed.

Homoeopathic Medicines

☞ For a nosebleed following an injury or trauma, give Arnica.

☞ For a bloody nose with a bright red face and a high fever, give Belladonna.

☞ If a child with a nosebleed has very pale cheeks, look at Ferrum phosphoricum.

☞ If the blood is dark, consider Hamamelis.

☞ For left sided nosebleeds with dark blood in a talkative person, consider Lachesis.

☞ If the person with the nosebleed asks for cold or carbonated drinks, look at Phosphorus.

Self Care and Home Remedies

Apply direct pressure by squeezing the sides of the nose shut with thumb and forefinger for five to ten minutes while breathing through the mouth.

Put a small piece of ice under the upper lip beneath the nose, or apply pressure to the point just under the nose on the upper lip.

Apply a cold compress to the nose.

2

Ayurvedic Cure of Disorders of Eyes, Ears and Nose

EYES STRAIN DUE TO TV WATCHING

- Boil ½ teaspoon fennel seeds (saunf) in a cup of water till it is reduced to half and cool it. Use as eye drops

Caution: Beware of contamination.

Eyes Tired

- Lavender oil offers gentle relief for tired and strained eyes. Add a drop of lavender oil to 500 ml (2½ cups) of water and shake the solution well. Dip two cotton wool pads in the liquid, squeeze out the excess water and place them over each eye. If you wear contact lenses, they must be removed before doing this.

Eyes Aching

When some foreign elements fall in your eyes, like the tiny bits of dust, even if they are removed the eyes ache. Another cause of it is lot of roaming about in the sun without use of the goggles.

- Boil a little of water a bowlful after adding just 10 gms. of turmeric to it. When cool, dip a clean soft cloth in this water, wrench the cloth midly to let a few drops go into your affected eyes. When water is pleasantly cool, throw this water on to your eyes and rub it dry by a soft towel. The pain will vanish soon.
- Put a drop of tulsi (Basil) juice mixed with even quantity of honey for a sort of eye troubles, especially

pain and burning. This solution can also be preserved in a bottle. If there be the problem of trachoma, grind ten leaves of tulsi together with a clove. Put it into your eyes after every four hours. If there, be swelling in the eyes, add a little of tulsi-juice with alum and apply in your eyes for instant relief.

- Powder equal quantities of liquorice (mulathi) and cumin (jeera). Take ½ teaspoon every day along with 1 teaspoon honey for a month.

Eyes Burning

- Mash 1 ripe banana along with a little curd and water, take twice a day.
- Mix equal quantities of fenugreek seed (methi daana) powder along with Shikakai powder for washing hair. Wash frequently.
- Grind an onion with 1 teaspoon each of black pepper and poppy seeds soak in ½ cup milk. Apply this paste on the head. Allow it to dry for 15-20 minutes. Wash with warm water.
- Mix the juice of bottle gourd and sesame oil (til ka tel) in the ratio of 4:1 and heat till the moisture is evaporated completely. Once cool, use it for massaging the head.

Eyes Sore

- Take a large lemon (bijora or galgal), make a whole into it and put a piece of turmeric in this cavity. In just two weeks time the lemon would be derived up and the turmeric piece would have sucked its juice. Now dry the turmeric in shade and grind it finely so that it may be strained through a fine cloth. Turn up the eyelids having this sore and rub lightly this powder. In just two days, all the eye sores will be cured and your eyes will become normal.

Cataract

The beginning of the cataract formation in the eye results in the sight failing. The affected one feels as if he is seeing through a glass. The cataract continues to get matured and the sight continues to fall. When it is fully mature. it is removed by surgical operation.

- Take 10 gms. of the juice of onions, good quality of honey 10 gms, and Bhimseni camphor (kapoor) 2 gms. Make a homogeneous mixture of the three and preserve them in a bottle. Every night before you go to sleep, apply it in your eyes by a eye liner. Its regular use prevents the cataract formation.

Cataract, Early Stage

- Mix 1 teaspoon rose water (gulab jal) with 1 teaspoon fresh lime juice. Add 10 drops of this to the eyes.
- Extract the juice of tulsi and add a little of honey to it. Apply this over the eyes every morning and evening. If the cataract be of raw type, it shall be cut away and if it be of ripe type, it shall be ripened soon to enable the doctor to remove it by operation.

Eyesight Failing

Take equal quantity of turmeric and the soft neem sprouts. Grind both of them in a handy stone crusher with the milk of the peepal added to it. Grind the lot for five days, pouring in fresh peepal milk everyday. From the 7th day onwards you can start using this paste like collyrium to line your eyes with. In just four weeks time your eye sight will not only stop fall. it will begin to improve as much as to make your reading glasses redundant.

- Stop reading at all in dim light or reading while lying down. Don't have very hot or very cold drinks. Eat easily digestible and nourishing food. Keep your bowels clean. Use the following powders:

- Take cumin seeds and coriander seeds in equal measure and sieve through a thin. clean cloth. Then take "Khand" in equal measure and grind the three again to a powdered from. Have about 10 gms. of this powder everyday in the evening and morning with fresh water. Wash your eyes with cold, clean water.

Eyesight Weakness

- Mix seeds of cardamom (chhoti illaichi) along with 1 tablespoon honey. Eat every day.
- Boil 2 tablespoons fenugreek (methi) leaves along with 1/2 cup moong dal and 10 small onions and eat regularly.
- Mix equal quantities of fenugreek seeds (methi daana) powder along with shikakai powder for washing hair. Wash your hair frequently.

Dark Circles Around Eyes

- Take one teaspoon tomato juice, 1/2 teaspoon lemon juice, a pinch of turmeric (haldi) powder and a little gram flour (besan). Make a paste and apply. Leave for 10 minutes and wash off.
- Drink tomato juice with a few mint leaves, little lemon juice and salt.
- Soak cotton wool in cucumber (kheera) or potato juice and apply around the eyes. You will find a change in 2-3 weeks.

Night Blindness

- The patients of this disease can't see anything in the dark. It can be caused by prolonged fever or continued undernourishment. Normally this trouble surfaces at the end of the rainy season. If it is not cured in six months time, it becomes rather chronic.
- The basic line of remedy is to feed the patient on easily digestible but nourishing diet. Regular use of milk

butter cream, half boiled eggs, green vegetables and fresh sweet vegetables are very effective to fight this ailment. If the constipatory tendency is there then administering the Murabba of 'Harh' together with 25 gms. of gulkand is very effective. Dropping the onion juice in the effected eyes for about a week (just two drops twice daily is very effective.

OTHER EYE TROUBLES

Eye wounds

Take a thick piece of turmeric and grind it on a clean stone like you grind sandalwood. Take this paste on your eye liner and put it in your eyes. The wounds will heal up soon. After applying this special paste, wash your eyes with lukewarm water after half an hour of the application. In the night, when you go to sleep, dip a cloth piece in turmeric boiled water after cooling it, and wrench the cloth to pour few drops every night over the eyes before you retire to bed. You can keep the cloth over your eyes for better relief.

Eye Web

- Boil about half kg. water with a pinchful of alum and half spoonful turmeric powder added to it. Now cool this water. Drench a cloth piece in this water and put it over your eyes. When this water is bearable warm, wrench this cloth to drop few drops of this water direct into your eyes. Do so in the evening and morning. In about ten days' time the webs will be dissolved.

Eye Pupil Outgrowth (Phuli)

- Take a heavy piece of turmeric, 10 gms. dry leaves of neem and 10 grams of black pepper. Grind them in a kharal after mixing adequate quantity of cow's urine.
- Everyday add fresh urine of cow and continue grinding it for six days. On the seventh day, add a little of

rose water and a piece of camphor. Now your surma is ready. Keep it as it is for three days more and start to line your eyes with the surma every evening and morning. Soon the outgrowh will be dissolved and your eye sight will also improve.

Trachoma

In this trouble the upper eyelid has some protruding growth which hurt the eye, causing it to grown and full of irritation.

- *Remedy:* Take 'rasout' 10 gms. Turmeric 3 gms. alum 3 gms, rose water 10 gms—soak all of them in a glass vessel overnight. And in the morning strain the solution through a thick cloth. Then fill in your eyes with the help of a dropper. In a week's time the trouble will vanish.

Eyes Oozing water voluntarily

This is a common ailment in which without any apparent trouble eyes continue to shed water.

- *Remedy:* Take 2 rattis of alum and dissolve it in a tola (a little more than 10 gms.) of rose water, soak cotton wad in this solution and put it over the eyes at least twice daily preferably first in the morning and then when you retire to bed.

Ear, Boils Inside

- Heat 2 teaspoons mustard oil. Add ½ teaspoon carom (ajwain) seeds and one or two flakes of crushed garlic (lahasun). Boil till they turn red. Filter it. Use as ear drops.

Ear Pain Due to Boils

- Heat 1 teaspoon each of garlic (lahasun) and carom seeds (ajwain) in 2 teaspoons mustard oil. When the garlic becomes brown, remove the oil from fire and cool it. Pour two drops in the aching ear.

- If there is swelling in the ears, then add the juice of bhanga with the juice of black tulsi and put a few drops of this juice inside the affected or both the ears for quick relief.

Ear Infections

- Extract 1 teaspoon juice from mango leaves. Slightly warm and use as ear drops when bearably hot.

Earache

- Heat 2 teaspoons mustard oil. Add ½ teaspoon carom seeds (ajwain) and one or two flakes of crushed garlic (lahasun). Boil till they turn red, filter it. Use as ear drops.
- Boil well 1 teaspoon lahasun (garlic) in 2 tablespoons ginger oil (til ka tel). Cool and filter. Use as ear drops (1 to 3 drops).
- Mix a few drops of lime juice in 1 teaspoon lukewarm water. Put 4 drops of this into the ear.
- Use neem leaves juice as ear drops.
- Take radish leaves, put them in 25 gms. of mustard oil and cook it slowly. Boil them as much as to reduce the watery content of the leaves to naught . When cold, strain and put it in a clean bottle. First of all, dip a cotton bud in this oil and clean your ears with it. Then drop a few drops of this oil. It is better if you do it by night when you retire to bed.
- Take about 10 leaves of makoy and ten leaves of tulsi. Extract their juice together and put it in the affected ear when it is slightly lukewarm (heat it a little in the sun). Alternatively add half a tablet of camphor in tulsi juice and put this juice in the ear for instant relief.
- If lukewarm basil leaves juice is dropped in the affected ear, this remedy brings immediate relief.

- Take out the juice of marigold flower's leaves, heat it a little and put it just two drops at a time twice daily.
- Take out the extract of beetroot leaves, heat it a little and drop just two to three drops in the affected ear.
- Make water saline by dissolving 'Sendha Namak' into it. Put a few drops daily morning and evening.
- Mix honey in the ginger juice with salt. Heat it a little and put two drops in the affected ear.

Ear Oozing Fluid

- 20 gms. of alum, turmeric 1 gm. grind both of them to a fine powder form and keep the powder in the bottle. Before using the powder, clean the ear thoroughly with a cotton wad. Then get this powder blown in the affected ear just 5 gms., of it every time. A few days regular use will cure the trouble.
- Heat a bit the juice of onion and drop two drops of it in the affected ear. This is an ideal remedy for all the ear troubles.

Ear Trouble (Pus Formation)

- To clear out the pus, take two pieces of turmeric and roast them in the mustard oil. Now strain the oil and fill it in a clean bottle. Pour either a few drops of this oil into the ear or clean the inside with the help of cotton buds dipped in this oil. In a fortnight the pus formation will stop and your hearing power shall be also enhanced.

Deafness

If the trouble is congenital or caused by some external injury, it can't be cured. But if it is caused by some internal disturbance in the ear, then it can certainly be cured by the following treatment:

- Take a sallow leaf of the plant of swallow worf. See that it has no holes. Heat it on fire a little and then extract its juice and drop it into the affected ear. About two weeks regular treatment can cure the ailment. Even the wound in the ear can also be cured by this treatment.
- Drop a few drops of lukewarm juice of onion into the ear. Onion juice is good for all the ear ailments. Even the similar use of bitter almonds can cure the ailment.
- Use raw onion juice as ear drops.
- Put two drops of lukewarm neem oil inside the ear.

Nose Blockage due to Cold and Phlegm

- Make into a very fine powder equal quantities of the following: green cardamom (chhoti illaichi) seeds, cinnamon (dalchini), black pepper (kali murch) and cumin seeds (jeera). Sniff this powder frequently to induce sneezing.

Nose Running

- Rub a nutmeg (jaiphal) on a smooth grinding stone along with some cow's milk. Apply this paste on forehead and nose.

Sneezing

- Boil 2 tablespoon fennel seeds (saunf) in 1 cup water till it is reduced to half. Filter it. Take 1 tablespoon every morning and evening for a few days.

Sinus

- Take a smokeless but burring cow dung cake and sprinkle turmeric powder over it. It will emit large quantities of smoke. Inhale this smoke deeply. It will release the stuck up solid phlegm in the nose and the patient will be cured.

Cold with Phlegm (Balgam) and Slight Cough

- Take 8-10 tulsi leaves and wash them well. In the 1 cup of water, add these tulsi leaves, 1-2 cloves of garlic (lahasun), ½ piece ginger, crushed and 4-5 peppercorns (saboot kali mirch). Boil the water and keep simmering on fire till the quantity is reduced to ¼ cup. Cool it. Strain the portion and add 1 teaspoon honey. Drink this every morning.

Nose Bleeding

- Take a big piece of turmeric and grind it with half kilo of dried bansa leaves. Add 25 gms. rock salt. Boil the lot in water till the quantity is reduced one fourth of the original quantity. Strain the potion and cool it. Take just 10 gms. of it at one hourly interval just sip the potion. In a couple of hours the extra heat of the blood shall pass out with urine and the nose bleeding will stop. Externally make the patient smell a cotton wet with the itra of khus for quick relief.
- Drop lemon juice in nostrils.
- Use juice of fresh coriander leaves (dhania) as nasal drops.
- Dip a cotton bud in rosewater and dab it on to the inside of your nostrils to stop the bleeding.

Nose Bleeding due to Body Heat

- Lemon juice dropped into nostrils provides excellent relief.
- Juice of fresh coriander leaves (dhania) can be used as nasal drops.
- The easiest and most effective cure of this trouble is to keep the tulsi blossom near you and smell it as and when you like. For those who are chronic patient of this trouble, this simple treatment is very effective and cures the trouble almost totally. Drinking tulsi juice mixed with honey will also help and provide extra strength to the body.

- Take 10gms. of fuller's earth and keep it in a cup full of water. When the process of sedimentation has taken place, drink the water early in the morning from the cup.
- Take a little of dry 'Aanwala' and soak it in about 25 gms. of water. Sieve through a fine cloth and drink the strained water early in the morning. The remaining material should be grinded to a paste form and be applied over palate and forehead.
- Grind 'Majufal' to fine powdered form and ask the patient to smell it repeatedly. The bleeding from the nose shall stop.

Cold and Cough

- The chronic patients of this problem have their hair going untimely white. To stop the process and cure it, take 300 gms. of tulsi leaves dried in shade, 50 gms. of Dalchini, 100 gms. Tejpat, 200 gms. Saunff (anise seeds), 200 gms of small cardamom, Agiya 300 gms; Banfshaw 25 gms; red sandal 200gms. and Brahmi herb 200 gms. grind all these ingredients and strain them through a cloth. Now take 10 gms. of this powder, boil it in 500 gms. water and when just a cup of this water remains, add sugar and milk and drink it twice a day like you have tea. All these problems will vanish in a couple of days.
- A tablespoon of carom seeds crushed and tied up in a muslin cloth can be used for inhalation to relieve congestion/blocked nose.
- A similar small bundle carom seeds placed near the pillow of sleeping children relieves congestion.
- A teaspoon of cumin seeds is added to 1 glass of boiling water. Strain and simmer for a few minutes. Let it cool. Drink it 1-2 times a day. If sore throat is also present, add a few small pieces of dry ginger to the boiling water.

- Six pepper corns finely grind and mixed with a glass of warm water, sweetened with 5-6 batasha can be taken for a few nights.
- In the case of the acute cold in the head, boil 1 tablespoon pepper powder in a cup of milk along with a pinch of turmeric (haldi) and have once daily for at least 3 days.
- A lemon a day keeps the cold away. For a bad cold, the juice of two lemons in ½ a litre (2½ cups) of boiling water sweetened with honey, taken at bed time, is a very effective remedy.
- Have ginger (adrak) tea. Cut ginger (adrak) into 1-1½ pieces and boil with a cup of water. Give 8-10 boils. Strain, sweeten with ½ teaspoon sugar and drink hot.

Foul Smeling Nose

Many person have this trouble. It is due to stomach disorder of the person. The following treatment is found to be quite effective.

- Grind the bitter pumpkin to a paste form and extract its juice. Drop two three drops of this pumpkin juice in the patient's nose. If you don't get fresh bitter pumpkin then you can take already dried pumpkin and soak it in water overnight. Grind it to a paste form early in the morning and drop this paste's juice in the sufferer's nose every morning. Besides this treatment, try to keep your digestive system in perfect order.

Nasal Congestion

- Crush a fistful of carom seeds (ajwain) and tie up in a cotton napkin and place it near the pillow.
- Put 1 teaspoon cardamom (chhoti illaichi) seeds on burning coal and inhale the smoke.

Nasal Congestion in Children

- Crush a fistful of carom seeds (ajwain) and tie up in a cotton napkin and place it near the pillow.

3

Respiratory Tract Disorders

Respiration provides us oxygen which is necessary for our life. We should take care of our respiratory system.

COMMON COLD

The common cold is a viral infection associated with a large number of viruses that infect the nose, throat, and lungs.

Symptoms

Sore throat and stuffy nose, with a watery nasal discharge at first, then becoming thicker and coloured. A low grade fever and headaches are common. A loose or dry, hacking cough often occurs as the cold "goes into the chest," and may persist for up to several weeks.

Complications

Colds may be complicated by bacterial infections leading to sinusitis and ear infections, and may progress to bronchitis or infrequently pneumonia.

Homoeopathic Medicines

Duing the first twenty four hours of a cold with a high fever, choose between Aconite, Belladonna, and Ferrum phosphoricum.

If the symptoms fit Belladonna but it doesn't help use Ferrum phosphoricum.

Allium cepa is the most common medicine for colds in which the eyes and nose run or drip like a faucet.

Give Kali bichromicum if the main symptom is pressing pain in the sinuses and root of nose. The discharge will usually be thick, greenish-yellow, and stringy.

If the symptoms come on after overwork or anger, and if the person is very impatient and irritable, look at Nux vomica.

Pulsatilla is good for a ripe cold with thick yellow green discharge, changeable moods, and a whiny, clingy disposition.

Give Arsenicum album for a cold with a watery, irritating nasal discharge in a chilly restless person who seems anxious and needy.

People who need Mercurius are sensitive to both heat and cold, with yellow green mucus and bad breath.

Self Care and Home Remedies

☞ Drink two to four cups of hot ginger tea. Boil three slices of fresh ginger in two cups of water for fifteen minutes.

☞ Avoid dairy products, wheat, bananas and oatmeal because they increase mucus production.

☞ Vitamin C (500 mg every two hours, up to 3000 mg per day) in the first stage of the cold.

☞ Beta-carotene: 50,000 IU per day.

☞ Zinc: 30 mg per day.

☞ Zinc lozenges if there is a sore throat.

☞ Garlic capsules, two every four hours.

☞ Nasal wash with one-fourth teaspoon salt to one cup warm water once or twice a day. For the nasal wash, snuff a small amount of salt water from a cupped hand into the nostrils. Tilt your head back closing the throat, let the water drain into your mouth and spit it out.

FLU

Flu, or influenza is an acute illness caused by the body's response to viral infection by influenza viruses, types A, B, or C. It often comes in the form of epidemics in the winter.

Symptoms

People with the flu complain of headache, fever and chills, aching muscles and joints, fatigue, sore throat, and cough. There is less nasal secretion and more fatigue than with the common cold. Flu sufferers often feel "wiped out," and just want to stay in bed. Some influenza has a gastrointestinal component with nausea, vomiting and diarrhea.

Complications

Conventional medicine has no effective treatment for the flu. Babies and the elderly sometimes succumb to the flu if it is very severe or complicated by secondary bacterial infections, particularly pneumonia.

Homoeopathic Medicines

☞ If the flu is just starting and there are no definite symptoms yet, choose between Oscillococcinum (also called "Flu Solution") and Ferrum Phosphoricum.

☞ Oscillococcinum is available over the counter in many pharmacies, health food stores, and supermarkets, and is our first choice at this stage unless high fever and red cheeks are prominent symptoms.

☞ After symptoms have developed, consider Bryonia if all the symptoms are made worse by movement and the person is very irritable and thirsty.

☞ Think about Gelsemium if the person is dizzy, drowsy, droopy, and dull, feels totally exhausted, and is not thirsty.

☞ Consider Eupatorium if the person feels deep aching in the bones and muscles and feels like his bones are broken.

☞ Give Rhus toxicodendron when stiffness is the main symptom, and it is made worse by cold damp weather or exertion, and better by stretching or moving around for a while.

Self Care and Home Remedies
Rest

☞ Drink plenty of fluids.

☞ If it is an upper respiratory flu, follow suggestions for common cold.

COLD, COUGHS, BRONCHITIS, AND FEVER

Cough and Bronchitis

Acute bronchitis is an inflammation of the bronchial tubes of the lungs. It is often associated with a cold or upper respiratory infection, fever, sore throat, and a nasal discharge or postnasal drip. Although infection is the most common cause, it may also be caused by inhaling irritant substances, or it may be a complication of allergies and sinusitis. Bronchitis usually lasts three to five days, or up to several weeks.

Symptoms

Coughs may be dry or loose. The most common symptoms are a tickling feeling in the throat or chest, fits of uncontrollable coughing, excessive mucus, interrupted sleep due to the inability to lie down without coughing hoarseness and pain in the throat, chest or head.

Complications

Bronchitis may lead to pneumonia in serious cases. Patients with shortness of breath, weakness or exhaustion, persistent fever, and a thick yellow green, brown, or bloody mucus from the lungs should see a qualified homoeopath or other medical practitioner immediately.

Homoeopathic Medicines

If the cough is extremely loose and rattly, think first of Antimonium tartaricum, then of Ipecac and Pulsatilla.

☞ If the person feels parched and is worse from any movement, give Bryonia.

☞ For bronchitis with fits of coughing, look at Drosera, Hepar sulphuris, Spongia and Rumex.

☞ For dry, croupy coughs, think first of Spongia, Drosera and Hepar sulphuris.

☞ For coughs that come from a tickle in the pit of the throat look at Rumex.

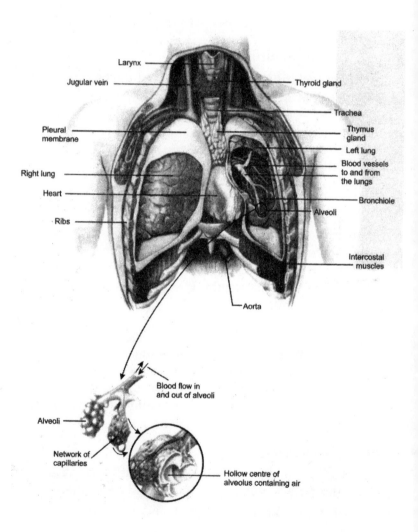

Self Care and Home Remedies

☞ For a wet cough, drink three to four cups a day of hot ginger tea. Boil three slices of fresh ginger in two cups of water for fifteen minutes.

☞ Hot water with plenty of freshly squeezed lemon juice and a little honey helps cut mucus. Drink three to four cups a day.

☞ Gargle with warm salt water.

☞ Vitamin C: 500 mg every four hours.

☞ Beta carotene: 50,000 IU per day.

☞ Zinc: 30 mg per day.

☞ Drink licorice root tea, one cup three times a day, as an expectorant.

☞ Avoid dairy products, sweets, and heavy foods.

Sinusitis

Sinusitis is an inflammation of the sinuses associated with viral, bacterial, or fungal infections or allergies.

Symptoms

The most common symptom is mild to severe pain in the maxillary or frontal sinuses. There may also be pain in the face or teeth. There is generally nasal discharge or stuffiness and often a sinus headache. It is the deep sinus pain that usually differentiates sinusitis from the common cold.

Complications

A severe bacterial sinusitis left untreated could potentially cause a more serious systemic infection.

Homoeopathic Medicines

☞ The first medicine to think of for sinusitis with pressing pain in the cheekbones and a thick, ropy nasal discharge is Kali bichromicum.

☞ If the sinusitis came after exposure to a draft, look first at Hepar sulphuris then at Nux vomica.

☞ If there are bad smelling odors in the nose and sinuses, think of Mercurius and Hepar sulphuris.

☞ If the sinusitis is much worse from going outdoors, think of Nux vomica and Hepar sulphuris.

☞ In a child with a sinus infection who is clingy, weepy, and moody, give Pulsatilla.

☞ If the sinusitis is much better from going outside, he probably needs Pulsatilla.

Self Care and Home Remedies

☞ Hot, moist packs applied to the sinuses can relieve congestion.

☞ Echinacea and goldenseal combination (two dropper-fuls of tincture in water three times a day or six capsules a day) is useful to stimulate the immune system to fight infection.

☞ Give Vitamin A (25,000 IU per day) or betacarotene (50,000 IU per day).

☞ Give Vitamin C (1000mg three times per day).

☞ Give Zinc (30 mg per day).

☞ Nasal irrigation with one quarter teaspoon of salt in one cup of warm water can be very helpful. Plastic or porcelain neti pots are a particularly effective way to accomplish this.

☞ Hot, spicy food such as cayenne, black pepper, and horse radish can help clear the sinuses.

☞ Avoid dairy products sweets, and cold and carbonated drinks.

☞ Boil four slices of fresh ginger root in a quart of water for fifteen minutes and drink three to four cups a day.

■

(4)

Ayurvedic Cure of Disorders of Respiratory System

COUGH (DRY)

- Nearly 250 gms. of sweet apples should be taken daily for a week to obtain relief.
- A glass of warm water with juice of 1 lime and 1-2 teaspoon of honey is very good for cough.
- Mix 8-10 tablespoons of coconut milk with 1 tablespoon poppy seeds (khuskhus) and 1 tablespoon pure honey. Take every night before going to bed.
- Mix equal amounts of honey and ginger (adrak) juice for better results, warm the mixture a little and then have it. Have 1 teaspon, 2-3 times a day.
- Three pepper corns (saboot kali mirch) sucked with a pinch of black cumin (shah jeera) and a pinch of salt gives relief.
- Mix 1 teaspoon pepper powder with 4 teaspoon gur (Jaggery). Make small balls. Suck 3-4 balls/tablets during the day.
- Mix equal amounts of pepper powder and sugar candy (mishri) by weight, mix enough pure ghee to form.
- Small balls. Suck one ball/tablet 3-4 times a day. Avoid-curd, bananas, ice, rice, fried and cold foods.
- Give 1 teaspoon of basil (tulsi) leaves juice, 2-3 times a day to children having cough. Tulsi leaves can be crushed to a paste and the paste squeezed through a clean muslin cloth to get juice.

- Mix a pinch of turmeric (haldi) with warm 1 cup milk and have at night.

WHOOPING COUGH

- Take about 10 gms. of tulsi leaves and even amount of black pepper. Now grind them together to homogeneous powder form. Now adding a little of honey to the combination and make small tablets. These astringent tasting tablets should be taken at least four times a day. Don't swallow these tablets but suck them slowly.
- If the accompanying cough be of dry type, add a little of honey then additionally, make the patient have the combined juice extracted from the even amount of tulsi seeds, ginger and onion. In case of wet cough add sugar candy also in the combination.
- Crush about 50 gms. of radish in your house and add equal amount of sugar cane juice. It would be advisable to add a piece of ginger's juice also in the concoction. Have this combination at least twice a day for speedier relief.
- Radish is a very tasty and useful vegetable and must form the part of everyone's diet. Another root, which is also full of medicinal qualities and equally tasty is carrot.

COUGH WITH PHLEGM (BALGAM)

- Mix equal amounts of onion juice and honey. Have 1 teaspoon 3-4 times a day. This is a preventive medicine against cold in winter.

Cought with Phlegm in Child

- A child suffering from this trouble should do away from all foods which produce phlegm like milk, ghee, sweets, rice, refined flour products, sugar and lentils. Give the child citrus but sweet fruits. Some tested remedies are given below:

- Burn the plantain leaves to ashes and ask the child to lick about 5 gms. of this ash daily. In about two weeks time this trouble shall be over.
- If the child is also afflicted with constipation, make him lick the combination of pure honey 6gms. and castor - oil 6 gms; followed by the combination of cumin seeds, liquorice, munnekka 3, boiled in water, mixed with pure honey.
- Chew a clove (laung) with a pinch of salt to ease expectoration and relieve irritation in throat.
- Pour 1 cup of boiling water over 1/2 teaspoon each of ginger powder, clove powder and cinnamon powder. Filter it. Sweeten with 1 teaspoon honey and drink.

ASTHMA

- Extract about 200 gms. of carrot juice and add about 100gms. of spinach juice with it. Have this combined juice at least thrice a day for getting relief. But one must continue this treatment at least for three months for its total cure. Have carrot and spinach also as salad in addition.
- An expectorant and a very effective remedy for asthma is prepared by boiling 6 cloves (laung) in 3 tablespoons of water. Take 1 teaspoon of this decoction with a little honey, thrice daily.
- Mix equal amounts of fresh ginger (adrak) juice, honey and pomegranate (annaar) juice. Take 1 tablespoon, 1-2 times a day.
- Figs are known to give relief by draining the phlegm (balgam). Take 3-4 dry figs, wash them well with warm water. Soak overnight in a cup of water. Eat them first in the morning and also drink the water. Do this for at least 2 months.
- Take 'Alshi' (10 gms) and after coarsely grinding it, boil in about 250 gms. of water. When water remains half

due to evaporation, add 20 gms. of honey to it. Honey is a very effective expectorant.

- Juice of onions 50 gms; the juice of gwarpathe 50 gms; ginger juice 50gms. and pure honey 10 gms. Mix them all in a glass container. Close it with the lid and dig it underground for 72 hours. Then take it out and let the patient lick it 6 gms. each time, at least twice daily, preferably in the morning and evening.
- If available then take indigenous wax, resin and ghee. Mix the three and put it over the live charcoal. The smoke emitted by the mixture should be inhaled deeply by the patient of asthma. This smoke clears the chest congestion and relieves the tension in the lungs.
- Mix 1 teaspoon honey with 1/2 teaspoon cinnamon powder and have it at night before going to bed.
- Boil carom seeds in water and inhale the steam.
- Boil 8-10 flakes of garlic (lahasun) in 1/2 cup of milk. Have this every night. It gives excellent results in early stages of asthma.
- Add a handful of drumstick leaves to 1 cup water. Boil, simmer on low flame for 3-4 minutes. Cool and strain. Add salt, pepper and lemon juice to taste. Have everyday, once or twice a day.
- Mix 1/4 teaspoon asafoetida, 2 teaspoons honey, 1/2 teaspoon juice from betel leaf (paan ka patta) 1/2 teaspoon white onion juice. Have it 2-5 times a day. To take out juice from betel, crush to a paste and squeeze through a clean muslin cloth. For onion juice, grate the onion and squeeze through a clean muslin cloth.

BREATHING PROBLEM

- Mix 1 teaspoon camphor (kapoor) in 1/2 cup slightly warm coconut oil and apply on the chest.

- Boil 2 tablespoon fennel seeds (saunf) in 1 cup water till it is reduced to half. Filter it. Take 1 tablespoon every morning evening for a few days.
- Boil 3 tablespoon powdered nutmeg (jaiphal) in 1 cup sesame oil (til ka tel). Cool it and apply on affected parts.
- Mix 1 teaspoon oil of garlic (lahasun) and 3 teaspoons honey and take a small amount three times a day.

PNEUMONIA

- Get the pure tulsi oil from a recognised Ayurvedic medicine shop. Put this oil on the chest of the afflicted person. Together with this treatment, extract the juice of five tulsi leaves, Mix it with a few grind grains of black peper at 6 hourly interval. This combined treatment will produce enough heat in the body to make the person sweat. With sweat all the effect of cold inside the body shall vanish and the patient will be cured.
- Take a thick cloth and make four folds of it. Between the third and fourth fold, spread a layer of turmeric. Now mix turmeric in lukewarm water and sprinkle over the cloth to make it partially wet. Now put this cloth on the chest of the patient, heat a brick and put it over the chest of the patient to foment his chest, when the heat from the brick reaches your chest, it would nullify the pneumonia effect. Also take one gm. of black pepper, five cloves and one gm. of edible soda. Boil it in 15 gms. of water. When it is drinkable, make the patient sip it for early relief.

CHEST CONGESTION

- Add to 1/2 litre of boiling water, 1 teaspoon carom seeds powder along with 1 teaspoon turmeric powder. Cool it and take 1 tablespoon of this mixture alongwith 1 teaspoon honey.

CHEST CONGESTION CAUSING BREATHING PROBLEM

- Grind 1/4 teaspoon mustard seeds (sarson) to a smooth paste. Mix with honey and eat.
- Mix equal quantities of mustard powder and rice flour. Add some water and boil until it reaches a paste like consistency. Spread on a handkerchief and foment the chest and neck when bearably hot.

■

Teeth and Digestive Disorders

Due to inaccurate eating practices, one can suffer from several digestive disorders.

Digestion of the food start from mouth itself with the help of Saliva. We should take care of our teeth for proper digestion.

TEETH DISORDERS

Teething

Some children have no problems at all when their first teeth break through. For others, it is quite an ordeal, and for their parents as well.

Symptoms

The most common symptoms of teething are pain in the teeth and gums, drooling, redness and swelling of the gums, fever, changes in the stool, restlessness, fussiness, and difficult sleeping.

Complications

Teething can be a challenging event, even though there are no complications.

Homoeopathic Medicines

☞ If the baby is chubby, contented, sweaty on the back of his head, and slow to teethe, give Calcarea carbonica.

☞ For babies who are beside themselves and inconsolable when they teethe and whose tantrums are outrageous, give Chamomilla.

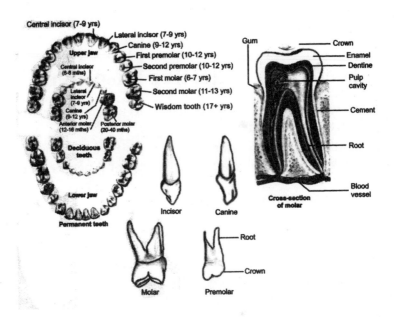

Central incisor (7-9 yrs)
Lateral incisor (7-9 yrs)
Canine (9-12 yrs)
Upper jaw
First premolar (10-12 yrs)
Central incisor (6-8 mths)
Second premolar (10-12 yrs)
First molar (6-7 yrs)
Lateral incisor (7-9 yrs)
Second molar (11-13 yrs)
Canine (9-12 yrs)
Wisdom tooth (17+ yrs)
Anterior molar (12-16 mths)
Posterior molar (20-40 mths)
Deciduous teeth
Lower jaw
Permanent teeth

Incisor   Canine

Molar   Premolar   Root   Crown

Gum   Crown
Enamel
Dentine
Pulp cavity
Cement
Root
Blood vessel
Cross-section of molar

☞ If she is peevish and nothing pleases her, but she's not as fussy as described for Chamomilla, give Calcarea phosphorica.

☞ If Calcarea phosphorica doesn't work, give Chamomilla.

☞ If the baby has delicate features, is constipated, and is slow to teethe, give Silica.

Self Care and Home Remedies

☞ Giving the baby something cold to chew on often relieves discomfort. This can be a pacifier or teething ring that has been put briefly in the freezer, or ice wrapped in a clean, wet cloth.

☞ If you cannot find homeopathic medicines, give the baby dilute chamomile tea.

☞ If you cannot find any single homoeopathic medicines and you are desperate, try the homeopathic combination teething tablets. (Biocombination No. 21)

TOOTHACHE

Pain in the teeth, sometimes involving the gums and mucous membranes.

Symptoms

The pain may range from mild to severe, and is often affected by chewing, hot and cold, and draft. Common causes of tooth pain are tooth decay, dental abscesses, nerve sensitivity, dental work, sinus infections, trauma, and damage to the facial nerve.

Complications

Complications include abscesses, death of a nerve (necessitating a root canal), loss of a tooth, or a severe, untreated infection that can become systemic.

Homoeopathic Medicines

☞ For very severe dental pain with great irritability, give Chamomilla or Hepar sulphuris.

☞ If drinking coffee aggravates the pain terribly, give Chamomila.

☞ For toothaches relieved by sloshing cold water in the mouth, give Coffea.

☞ If the pain is due to a very sensitive dental abscess, give Hepar sulphuris.

☞ If the toothache is accompanied by bad breath, a very coated tongue, and a lot of salivation, give Mercurius.

☞ If the toothache is unbearable and is limited to the left side of the face, consider Plantago.

Self Care and Home Remedies

☞ Ice may temporarily numb the pain.

☞ Clove oil acts as an analgesic, but may interfere with homoeopathic medicines.

☞ Take white willow bark or another pain reliever temporarily until the homeopathic medicines have a chance to act.

DIGESTIVE DISORDERS

Colic

Colic is a condition found in babies from just after birth until three or four months of age, with crying, irritability, and what seems to be pain or cramps in the abdomen. They usually seem quite hungry, eat and gain weight normally, and particularly like to suck. The actual cause and process by which colic happens are unknown.

Symptoms

Colicky babies cry and appear to be in pain or distress. Gas may be part of the problem. They may cry incessantly, or only

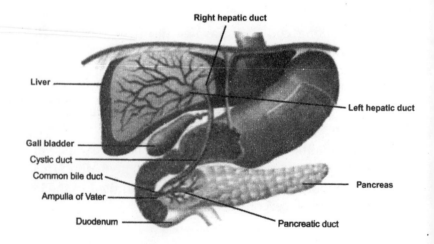

at certain times. The crying can be very distressing to parents, who feel helpless to do anything about it.

Complications

Simple colic is not life-threatening, not does it lead to any serious illness. It usually passes on its own in a matter of weeks. If the baby doesn't gain weight, vomits excessively, or has persistent diarrhea, medical attention should be sought to determine the cause of the problem.

Homoeopathic Medicines

☞ If the baby can't seem to tolerate milk, first think of Aethusa, then Magnesia phosphorica, Calcarea carbonica or Lycopodium.

☞ If there is a tendency toward frequent belching, and the baby seems to feel better after belching, Carbo vegetabilis is likely to be needed.

☞ For colic in extremely fussy, irritable babies, especially if they arch their backs and are inconsolable, consider Chamomilla.

☞ If a baby doubles over with the colic or brings his knees up to his chest, think of Colocynthis first then Magnesia phosphorica.

☞ For colic with excessive bloating and gas, particularly if the baby seems to be worse after ingesting milk, look at Magnesia phosphorica.

Self Care and Home Remedies

☞ Make sure the baby has been burped after eating.

☞ Rocking, carrying or holding the baby may soothe him.

☞ Gripe water is available in many East Indian grocery stores.

☞ Pacifiers may help with the uge to suck.

☞ Swaddling the baby fairly tightly and placing her on her stomach may help.

☞ A hot water bottle placed on the baby's abdomen may relieve discomfort.

AMEBIC DYSENTERY

Amebiasis is a parasitic infection caused by a microganism called Entamoeba bistolytica, more commonly known as amebas. It is usually contracted by ingesting cysts in drinking water or food contaminated with stool. It is more frequent in parts of the world where sanitation is poor, and is a problem often encountered by travelers to developing countries.

Symptoms

The main symptoms of amebic dysentery are painful abdominal cramps, loose watery stools, and gas. The stools may contain mucus and blood, and are infectious. amebas frequently cause liver swelling and tenderness and, less commonly, abscesses in the liver. The diagnosis is confirmed primarily by a laboratory examination of the stool called an "ova and parasite" test. Sometimes several stool samples are needed to find the amebas.

Complications

Since amebiasis may be confused with ulcerative colitis, irritable bowel syndrome, and other parasitic infections, diagnosis by a qualified medical professional is recommended. Dehydration, blood loss, and death are posible complications.

Homoeopathic Medicines

☞ If the person is extremely anxious and restless with diarrhea, give Arsenicum album.

☞ If the person has exhausting diarrhea with lots of cramping, think of Arsenicum album and Podophyllum.

☞ If the stool is explosive, consider Croton tiglium, Gambogia, or Podophyllum.

☞ If there is significant nausea and vomiting, first consider Ipecac, then Arsenicum album.

☞ If there is lots of rumbling and gurgling in the abdomen, give Podophyllum, Croton tiglium, or Gambogia.

☞ If there is profuse diarrhea and cramping with sweating and shivering, first think of Veratrum album then Arsenicum album.

Self Care and Home Remedies

☞ Drink plenty of fluids and replenish electrolytes, including sodium and potassium. Electrolyte solutions available from pharmacies are useful.

☞ Clear liquids such as water, vegetable broth, and diluted fruit juice help replace fluids.

☞ The diet should be light and bland; include vegetable soup, whole-grain toast, brown rice, bananas, and apple sauce.

☞ A warm pack over the abdomen is soothing and may reduce cramping.

☞ One tablespoon of psyllium seed husks per day often helps to firm up stools.

CONSTIPATION

Constipation means difficulty in passing stool, or the inability to have a bowel movement when desired. It can be caused by diseases affecting the bowel or nervous system, emotional stress, lack of bowel tone and peristalsis, insufficient fiber in the diet, dehydration, lack of exercise, drugs and, rarely, obstruction of the bowel.

Symptoms

Hard, dry, or soft stool, pain on having a bowel movement, gas and bloating and hemorrhoids are the main symptoms. Feelings of sluggishness, mental dullness, bad breath and body odor often accompany constipation.

Complications

Acute constipation mainly causes discomfort. If it persists, impaction of the hard, dry stool can occur, blocking the rectum and requiring manual removal. Enlargement of segments of the colon may occur if constipation is chronic and severe.

Homoeopathic Medicines

For constipation that is due to dryness with no urge, in a person who seems confused, consider Alumina.

☞ A person who needs Bryonia has large, hard stools with dryness, and a lot of thirst for cold drinks; many symptoms are worse from motion.

☞ For a stubborn, chilly flabby person who sweats on his head and has stubborn constipation, try Calcarea carbonica.

☞ When there is dryness, and a dreamy, drowsy, dizzy state, give Nux moschata.

☞ When the person is an irritable business person, consider Nux vomica or Bryonia.

☞ If the person has constant urges but can't go, even with a lot of straining, try Nux vomica.

☞ For constipation during pregnancy and menstruation, and a feeling like a ball in the anus of that the rectum and uterus will fall out, consider Sepia.

☞ For bashful stool (comes out part way, then recedes) in a refined, shy person with sweaty feet, try Silica.

Self Care and Home Remedies

☞ Drink eight glasses of water per day, starting with a glass of warm water with lemon immediately on rising in the morning.

☞ Eat lots of fresh fruits and vegetables, at least half of them raw.

☞ Eat whole grains and supplement with a tablespoon of bran stirred in juice or baked in muffins or in cereal.

☞ Take a one to three km. walk daily.

DIARRHEA

Acute diarrhea is usually due to infection by such bacteria as Staphylococcus, E. coli, Salmonella, or Shigella or such parasites as Amebas or Giardia lamblia. Infection may come from eating or drinking contaminated food or water. Some diarrhea is caused by emotional or digestive upset.

Symptoms

The stools are loose or watery, sometimes profuse or explosive and may be foul-smelling. Food particles may be found in the stool.

Complications

Diarrhea often results in loss of fluids and electrolytes such as sodium and potassium, which must be replaced to prevent dangerous levels of dehydration and electrolyte imbalance. Homeopathic medicines can stop diarrhea, but rehydration is still important.

Homoeopathic Medicines

☞ If stool is like jelly due to mucus, give Aloe.

☞ If the person is chilly, anxious, nervous and restless, Arsenicum album is your best bet.

☞ If diarrhea comes immediately after eating or drinking, look at Croton tiglium and Gambogia.

☞ If there is a lot of rectal itching with the diarrhea, combined with urgency first thing in the morning, Sulphur is indicated.

☞ If the diarrhea is violent and is accompanied by profuse sweating and chills, give Veratrum album.

Self Care and Home Remedies

Drink plenty of fluids and replenish such electrolytes as sodium and potassium. Electrolyte solutions available from pharmacies are useful. Clear liquids such as water, vegetable broth and diluted fruit juice help replace fluids.

The diet should be light and bland, including vegetable soup, whole grain toast, brown rice, bananas, and applesauce.

A warm pack over the abdomen is soothing and may reduce cramping. Calcium and Magnesium (500 mg per day) may also help to reduce cramping.

One tablespoon psyllium seed husks per day often helps to firm up stools.

HEMORRHOIDS

Hemorrhoids are varicose veins of the rectum. They may be inside the rectum, or they may protrude outward through the anus. They most commonly result from constipation or pregnancy, and may also be associated with liver problems.

Symptoms

The most annoying symptom associated with hemorrhoids is pain due to inflammation and swelling. This may range from a mild discomfort with or without itching, to pain so severe that sitting or having a bowel movement is excruciating. Hemorrhoids often bleed.

Complications

Blood clots may become lodged in the hemorrhoidal veins surrounding the hemorrhoid. The hemorrhoids may ulcerate and bleed profusely. Other possible causes of rectal bleeding should be investigated, including colitis, polyps and tumors.

Homoeopathic Medicines

    ☞ If the main symptom is pain like small sharp sticks in the rectum, consider Aesculus and Collinsonia.

☞ If swelling and bleeding are prominent, think first of Hamamelis..

☞ If the person is chilly, over stressed, and drinks too much alcohol, consider Nux vomica.

☞ In a warm blooded person with lots of the rectal itching and recal spasms, give Sulphur.

Self Care and Home Remedies

☞ Take a sitz bath. Fill the bathtub with hot water to two inches below the navel. Sit with knees bent. Stay in the tub for five minutes. Then squat in a tub of cold water for one minute. Repeat the cycle to three times.

☞ Take 1000 milligrams of bioflavonoids daily to strengthen the capillaries.

☞ Keep the rectal area clean.

☞ If you are constipated, drink plenty of water and take one tablespoon of bran, flaxseed oil, or psyllium seed one to two times daily until the constipation is relieved.

☞ Avoid spicy foods, they may aggravate the hemorrhoids.

☞ Get exercise to increase circulation in the pelvic area.

☞ Peel a garlic clove, scratch its surface several times and insert in the rectum as a suppository. Remove after eight hours or when the stool is passed.

HEPATITIS

Hepatitis is an inflammation of the liver, usually of viral origin, but it may also be caused by drugs or alcoholism. Hepatitis A is transmitted by contact with contaminated water or food, stool, blood, or secretions. Hepatitis B is transmitted primarily through blood transfusions or contaminated needles. Hepatitis C occurs mostly after blood transfusions, causing acute hepatitis that may become chronic. Legally it is necessary to call the local health department to report a newly diagnosed case of hepatitis.

Symptoms

Overall weakness or discomfort, nausea and vomiting, diarrhea, poor appetite, and fever are the main symptoms. Jaundice may be marked, depending on the stage of the hepatitis. Hives and joint pains may also occur.

Complications

Hepatitis causes severe liver dysfunction with jaundice, bloating, and diarrhea, and may be fatal in extreme cases. Hepatitis may become chronic, causing long term liver damage that can be fatal.

Homoeopathic Medicines

- ☞ The most common medicines are Chelidonium, china and Lycopodium.
- ☞ If there is considerable right shoulder blade pain, give Chelidonium.
- ☞ If the person has a history of gonorrhea or chlamydia, he probably needs Natrum sulphuricum.
- ☞ If perspiration and the breath smell bad and there is excessive saliva, give mercurius.
- ☞ If the person has a strong craving for cold drinks, look at Phosphorus.

Self Care and Home Remedies

- ☞ Get a hepatits screen to determine the type of hepatitis you have.
- ☞ Make sure that the local public health department has been contacted.
- ☞ Eat a light, low-fat diet with lots of fruits and vegetables, especially beets.
- ☞ Take Vitamin C, 1000 mg three times a day.
- ☞ Take liver herbs, including danelion root, milk thistle, or beet greens.

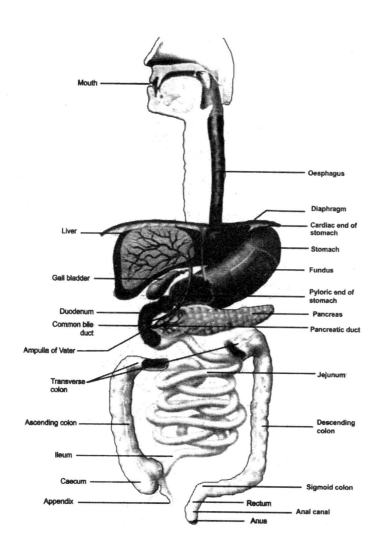

- Mouth
- Oesphagus
- Diaphragm
- Cardiac end of stomach
- Liver
- Stomach
- Fundus
- Gall bladder
- Pyloric end of stomach
- Duodenum
- Pancreas
- Common bile duct
- Pancreatic duct
- Ampulla of Vater
- Transverse colon
- Jejunum
- Ascending colon
- Descending colon
- Ileum
- Caecum
- Sigmoid colon
- Appendix
- Rectum
- Anal canal
- Anus

INDIGESTION AND HEARTBURN

Indigestion and heartburn are common conditions following eating too much or not being able to digest food properly.

Symptoms

Indigestion can include nausea, gas, belching, stomach pain, and heart burn. It usually occurs in the two hours immediately after eating. Heart burn is burning pain in the chest behind the sternum, which is associated with the reflux of acidic or caustic stomach fluids into the esophagus. Heartburn may occur after eating any food which stimulates acid production in the stomach, such as proteins, spicy foods, or chocolate.

Complications

Indigestion and heartburn are usually uncomplicated, and respond easily to change in diet, antacids, or homoeopathic treatment. The symptoms may be confused with symptoms of a stomach ulcer, a hiatal hernia, or angina. If indigestion is severe or persistent, medical attention should be sought to determine the cause of the problem.

Homoeopathic Medicines

- ☞ When extreme burnig pain is the main symptom, along with a lot of anxiety and restlessness, think of Arsenicum, especialy in a self-centered person who wants support and has many fears.
- ☞ Lycopodium is the medicine if the person is insecure yet bossy and full of false bravado, gets lots of gas from just a little food, and is worse from 4:00 to 8:00 P.M.
- ☞ When the person is irritable, impatient and hard-driving, and suffers from too much rich food, coffee and alcohol, give Nux vomica.
- ☞ Conversely, when the person suffers from rich food, but is mild, gentle, changeable and weepy and wants to be taken care of, think of Pulsatilla.
- ☞ If the person is lazy, intellectual, egotistical and sloppy and suffers from heartburn and morning diarrhea, give Sulphur.

Self Care and Home Remedies

- ☞ Avoid overeating, especially heavy or rich foods.
- ☞ Avoid fats, spicy foods, alcohol, coffee, and chocolate.
- ☞ Commercial antacids may provide temporary relief.
- ☞ Charcoal capsules are helpful in relieving gas. Take two capsules every four hours.
- ☞ Lying on the back and bringing the knees to the chest may cause gas to pass.
- ☞ Squatting helps gas to pass.
- ☞ Eliminate gas producing foods from the diet, such as beans, potatoes, sweets, and carbonated drinks.

NAUSEA AND VOMITING

Nausea and vomiting are symptoms of digestive distress that can come from many causes, including strong odors, morning sickness, motion sickness, food poisoning, indigestion, intestinal obstruction, alcohol intoxication, drug use, prescription drugs, chemotherapy, and exposure to toxic materials, as well as emotional causes such as anxiety, stage fright, and disgust.

Symptoms

Nausea is uneasiness of the stomach with a feeling that retching or vomiting might follow. Vomiting is the forcible emptying of the stomach contents through the esophagus and mouth. Vomiting may occur as single or repeated spasms which the body uses to empty the stomach. Unfortunately, vomiting may continue as dry heaves even after the stomach is empty if the stimulus is strong enough. In projectile vomiting, the stomach contents are ejected in a forcible stream that may extend for several feet.

Complications

Nausea and vomiting may lead to serious dehydration and possibly malnutrition if prolonged. Dehydration may require intravenous fluids if the person is unable to keep liquids down for more than a day.

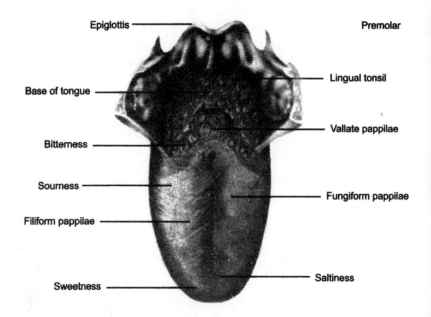

Homoeopathic Medicines

☞ Ipecac is the first medicine to think of for strong nausea and vomiting.

☞ Use Bismuth or phosphorus when the vomiting is primarily of liquids, and they are vomited after becoming warm in the stomach.

☞ Nux vomica should be considered when the vomiting comes on from emotional stress, especially anger and frustration, and it is difficult for the person to vomit.

☞ Phosphorus can be considered for vomiting blood and for vomit that looks like coffee grounds, in a friendly, open, sympathetic person who desires cold drinks but vomits them.

☞ Tabacum is the best for deathly nausea and vomiting from motion, like seasickness.

☞ Veratrum album is useful for a combination of nausea, vomiting, and diarrhea, especially if the person is very cold but desires ice and sour foods such as lemons and pickles.

Self Care and Home Remedies

☞ Get some fresh air.

☞ Eat small amounts of food frequently.

☞ Eat Saltine crackers to help relieve the nausea.

☞ Eat bland foods such as broth, rice, and pasta.

☞ Tea and toast are usually well tolerated.

☞ Drink clear fluids if you can keep them down.

☞ Sip ginger root tea to help relieve nausea. Use a one quarter inch slice of ginger root boiled in a cup of water for fifteen minutes.

☞ Stimulate Stomach an acupressure point in the soft place below the knee and to the outside of the leg where the tibia and fibula bones meet, to relieve nausea. Use firm rotary pressure on the spot for a few seconds. Repeat when needed.

STOMACH AND ACUTE ABDOMINAL PAIN

Stomach and abdominal pain can range from mild discomfort to incapacitating pain. The causes are highly variable and include indigestion, gas, appendicitis, gall bladder inflammation, liver problems, menstrual cramping, acute gastroenteritis, ectopic pregnancy, miscarriage, cancer, and anxiety, as well as a number of other causes.

Symptoms

Symptoms include localised or referred pain or cramping, nausea with or without vomiting, constipation or diarrhea, gas, bloating, abnormal stools, and other symptoms of anxiety, including rapid heartbeat and pulse, and perspiration.

Complications

Many complications can occur, depending on the source of the pain. A thorough workup by a gastroenterologist should be done for persistent or significant stomach or abdominal pain. If the pain is severe or incapacitating, emergency medical care should be sought to rule out life-threatening emergencies such as appendicitis, a gall bladder attack, or an ectopic pregnancy.

Homoeopathic Medicines

☞ If the stomach or abdominal pain is aggravated by motion, give Bryonia.

☞ If doubling up relieves the pain, think of Colocynthis or Magnesia phosphorica.

☞ The first medicine to think of for violent cramping is Cuprum.

☞ If the pain is relieved by standing up straight and made worse by bending double, the best medicine is Dioscorea.

☞ If the person gets bloated after eating even a small amount of food, choose Lycopodium.

☞ If pressure relieves the pain, consider Magnesia phosphorica, but if pressure aggravates the pain, look at Lycopodium.

☞ For stomach or abdominal pain after too much alcohol or spicy or rich foods, first think of Nux vomica.

☞ A plump, gentle, moody woman who doesn't do well with rich foods is likely to need Pulsatilla.

Self Care and Home Remedies

☞ Charcoal absorbs gas. If there is painful gas, give two charcoal capsules every two to four hours as needed.

☞ Peppermint or fennel tea can soothe indigestion.

☞ Castor oil packs applied for one hour with a heating pad can sometimes relieve abdominal distress.

☞ Avoid overeating, especially heavy or rich foods.

☞ Avoiding fats, spicy foods, alcohol, coffee, and chocolate may be helpful.

☞ Commercial antacids may provide temporary relief.

☞ Lying on the back and bringing the knees to the chest may cause gas to pass.

☞ Applying a heating pad to the area can help relieve pain.

GAS

Gas is a byproduct of fermentation or rotting of food in the digestive tract by yeast and bacteria. It may be odorless or foul smelling. Fermentation produces carbon dioxide, which has no smell. Bacteria often produce methane and hydrogen sulfide, which do have a foul smell.

Symptoms

Belching, passing gas and abdominal bloating with rumbling sounds are the most common symptoms of gas.

Complications

Gas may be painful if it is trapped in the stomach or intestines. More serious abdominal problems are sometimes mistaken for simple gas pains. If gas doesn't resolve within six to twelve hours, or is very severe or accompanied by fever, nausea, and vomiting, seek medical attention to get a proper diagnosis of the abdominal pain.

Homoeopathic Medicines

☞ If bloating is extreme or if the person is exhausted or collapsed and wants to be fanned, give Carbo vegetabilis.

☞ If the person is doubled over in pain and doubling over makes him feel better, give Colocynthis.

☞ When gas and bloating take away the appetite, and the person lacks confidence and is worse from 4:00 to 8:00 pm., give Lycopodium.

☞ If the person is chilly, irritable and impatient and can't seem to pass the gas without straining, give Nux vomica.

☞ When the person is weepy, changeable and clingy and has eaten too much fat or rich food, give her Pulsatilla.

Self Care and Home Remedies

☞ Charcoal capsules are helpful in relieving gas. Take two capsules every four hours.

☞ Lying on the back and bringing the knees to the chest may cause gas to pass.

☞ Squatting helps relieve gas.

☞ Massaging the abdomen in a clockwise direction helps the lower bowel gas to pass.

☞ Babies may be burped over the shoulder.

☞ Treat constipation to relieve chronic gas.

☞ Eliminate gas forming foods from the diet., such as beans, potatoes, sweets, and carbonated drinks.

6

Ayurvedic Cure of Disorders of Mouth, Throat and Teeth

SORE THROAT

- Apply liquorice mulathi paste around the throat for relief.
- Eat a plain betel leaf (pan) with liquorice (mulathi) 2-3 times a day.
- Drink tea boiled with ginger (adrak) and a few tulsi leaves 2-3 times a day.
- Gargle with warm salt at least twice a day. However do not make gargling sounds as this may aggravate the soreness.
- Pound 2-3 cloves (laung), garlic (lahasun) and add to a cupful of honey. Keep for 1-2 days, have one teaspoon thrice a day.
- Drink lots of water (10-12 glasses) everyday, since most throat problems are intensified by dehydration.
- Have the mixture of ½ teaspoon honey and ½ teaspoon lemon juice every 1-2 hours.

Throat Pain

- Crush a few neem leaves with water. Remove pulp. Warm it up. Add a little honey and gargle three or four times a day.
- Mix 1 teaspoon lime juice and 1 tablespoon honey. Swallow tiny amounts slowly 2-3 times a day.

Throat Hoarseness

- Soak 8 to 10 almonds overnight in 1 cup of water. After discarding the outer skin, grind the kernels with 8 to 10 black pepper (saboot kaali mirch) in 1 cup of water. Sift it and drink once a day, after adding sugar candy (mishri) to taste.
- Take 1 teaspoon onion juice mixed with 1 teaspoon honey.
- Pour 1 glass boiling water on a mixture of 1 teaspoon each of crushed cinnamon sticks (dalchini) and green cardamoms (chooti illaichi). Keep aside. Filter and use as a gargle when warm.
- Boil 2 teaspoons fennel seeds in barley water and take twice or thrice a day.

Hoarse Voice

- Mix seeds of green cardamom (chhoti illaichi) along with 1 tablespoon honey. Eat everyday.
- Add 2 tablespoon of fenugreek seeds to 6 cups of water. Heat on low flame for 15-20 minutes. Cool to bearable temperature. Strain and gargle with this, 2-3 times a day.
- Heat a cup of milk till warm. Add 1-2 pinches of turmeric powder (Haldi), mix well and drink at night.
- Just extract the juice of 10 tulsi leaves, add a little of honey and lick it. Just a small spoon full quantity of this solution will soothe your throat nerves and your voice will be again sweet.

Mouth Infection

- Powder dried mint (pudina). Use as toothpowder.

Mouth Inflammation

- Soak 1 tablespoon crushed liquorice (mulathi) root in 2 cups of water for 2 to 3 hours and use it for gargling frequently.

Bad Odour

- Use neem twigs as toothpaste.
- Powder the dried mint (pudina) leaves. Use as tooth-powder.
- Boil some cinnamon (dalchini) in a cup of water. Store it in a clean bottle in your bathroom. Use it as a mouth wash frequently.
- Parsley leaves are rich in chlorophyll, nature's own deodoriser. Chew some leaves regularly and your breath will remain fresh. Alternatively, you can chew some cardamom seeds (illaichi) to sweeten your breath. Chew some fennel seeds frequently.
- Chew a piece of cinnamon (dalchini) put in a betel leaf (paan ka patta).
- Tea made by boiling 1 teaspoon fenugreek seeds (methi dana) taken twice or thrice a day. A little honey or lemon juice can be added to improve the flavour.

Mouth Ulcers (Apathae)

- Chew one or two tender leaves of fig (angeer) and leaf buds frequently and wash the mouth with warm water.
- Soak 1 tablespoon crushed liquorice (mulathi) root in 2 cups of water for 2 to 3 hours and use it for gargling frequently.
- Boil 2 tablespoons fenugreek (methi) leaves along with ½ cup green gram (saboot moong dal) and 10 small onions. Eat regularly.
- Fenugreek seeds (methi dana), fried and powdered. This is added to drinking water. Drink 2-3 times daily for 2-3 days.
- Pour boiling water over fenugreek (methi) leaves. Keep aside till lukewarm. Strain and gargle with this infusion, 5-6 times daily for a couple of days.
- Mix some coconut milk with honey and massage the gums 3 to 4 times a day.

- Gargle with (or apply) freshly extracted coconut milk from a ripe coconut frequently.
- Mix the pulp of a ripe bel fruit with jaggery (gur) and eat once a day.
- Mix tea cup bel pulp with 1 teaspoon sugar and eat early morning on an empty stomach for 3 days.
- Prepare coriander (dhania) decoction by boiling 1 teaspoon coriander seeds (saboot dhania) in 1 cup of water and gargle frequently, when lukewarm.

Mouth Boils

- Take just a leaf of Chameli plant, and four leaves of tulsi. Chew them properly for a few minutes and suck in the juice. In about a day the trouble will vanish.

Teeth Disorders

- Teeth are very vital factors in the process of digestion because it is they which first deal with the food one eats. These teeth are of quite different varieties. Some cut the food, some munch it and some press it with the help of saliva. Teeth are important not only to help indigestion but also to keep the face beautiful.

Toothache and Infirmity of Teeth

- Take 10 gms. of pippali churna, Sendha namak 10 gms, grind them to a powdered form and use this combination as the tooth powder to clean your teeth.
- In case of toothache, rub a little of honey over your teeth and allow the saliva to flow out of the mouth. If your teeth has a worm or cavity then fill it with the above mentioned powder and then rinse your mouth.
- Take ammonium chloride 5 gms. and put it by means of a cotton wad to the affected teeth. Allow saliva to ooze out. The toothache shall vanish soon.

- Heat 1 teaspoon coconut oil and fry 3 pieces of cloves (laung) powder. Apply on the affected area.
- Apply nutmeg oil in affected parts.
- Burn the shells of almonds and powder it. Use as tooth-powder.
- Soak a piece of cotton wool in a few drops of clove oil. Press on affected areas.
- Paste of dry ginger (saunth) applied to gums alongwith a little salt.
- Apply a mixture of powdered black pepper (kali mirch) and clove oil on the affected part.
- Pound some asafoetida (heeng) in a mortar and pestle and add some lime juice. Heat it slightly. Soak a piece of cotton and hold it on the affected area.
- Take 3 gms of turmeric, 3 cloves and three dried leaves of guava. Boiling them in 250 gms. of water and after straining it through a fine sieve, rinse your mouth with this lukewarm water for about 15 minutes. You could get instant relief. Alternatively, roast a turmeric piece in hot ash and then press the turmeric by your aching teeth. Do so for two minutes and then the saliva come out of your mouth. Spit it away. Soon the trouble will vanish.

Teeth Weakness

- Burn to ashes a piece of turmeric, grink it with Bishop's weed (ajwain) and use this mixed powder as your tooth powder. Continuing cleaning your teeth with this powder would provide relief in a couple of week's time. When you apply this powder to your teeth, allow the saliva to ooze out for a few minutes before rinsing your mouth. But, avoid taking very hot drinks and stop consuming sweets in excessive quantity. Sweets especially the white cleaned sugar is very bad for the teeth, just avoid it.

Tooth Decay

- Take a piece of turmeric, roast it and then grind it to powder form. Then fill this powder in the cavity caused by tooth decay. In case you are unable to sleep owing to toothache caused by the decay in teeth or tooth, then grind turmeric, bishop's weeds and cloves and tie them in a small piece of cloth. Put this cloth below the aching teeth press it mildly and let the teeth get the essence of these ingredients. As you ooze the saliva out your toochache will vanish with it.

Tooth Yellow

- Mix salt with finely powdered rind of lime (nimbu ka chilka). Use this as toothpowder frequently.
- Burn the shells of almonds and powder it. Use as toothpowder.

Filthy Teeth

- Burn an oyster shell to ashes, add a little of salt, grind and sieve through a fine cloth and preserve the powder for rubbing it over the teeth.
- Take about 50 gms, of keekarwood, roasted alum 20 gms and namak lahori 10 gms, grind and sieve the whole mixture and rub this powder over your teeth every morning and evening.

■

7

Kidney/Urinary Bladder and Joint Disorders

We should drink plenty of water for proper cleaning of our excretory system. We should consume in less quantity foods such as tomato, brinjal, spinach, if we are suffering from any kidney or urinary bladder disorder.

BLADDER INFECTIONS

Bladder infections are caused by microorganisms that colonise the bladder in susceptible patients. Bladder infections may have no apparent symptoms even though bacteria can be cultured from the urine. Symptoms may also occur with no apparent infection.

Symptoms

The most common symptoms are urgent desire to urinate, frequent urination, bladder pain, low back pain, and burning pain before, during or after urination. Bladder infections occur most commonly in women following sexual intercourse, especially with a new partner. Bladder infections can also occur after waiting too long without urinating or going too long without drinking liquids. Catheterisation is a common source of bladder infections in hospitals and nursing homes. Bladder infections often come on with sudden severity, but can progress gradually.

Complications

There is risk of bladder infections ascending up the ureter to cause acute pyelonephritis, a serious infection of the

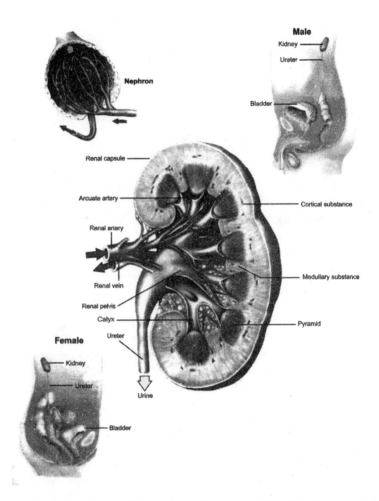

kidneys. Pain along the sides of the mid-back along with urinary frequency, urgency, and pain is indicative of a kidney infection and requires immediate treatment.

Homoeopathic Medicines

- ☞ The most common medicines for bladder infections are Cantharis and Staphysagiria.
- ☞ Think of Apis if the pain is mostly stinging and burning, there is any swelling, the last drops feel scalding, and the urine will not come out easily.

☞ Give Cantharis if blood in the urine is prominent or the pain is excruciating. Cantharis has the most extreme bladder symptoms.

☞ If the major symptom is frequent, intense urging with very severe pain, give Mercurius corrosivus.

☞ Sarsaparilla is a very common medicine for women's bladder infections.

☞ If the major symptom is burning in the urethra at the close of urination, give Sarsaparilla. If it doesn't work, look at Staphysagria or Cantharis.

☞ If the bladder infection comes on after sex, consider Staphysagria first.

Self Care and Home Remedies

☞ Drink as much water as possible.

☞ Urinate whenever you have the urge.

☞ Avoid horseback riding or other activities that put pressure on the urethra and bladder.

☞ Take bladder herbs such as Oregon grape, Buschu, Pipsissewa, and Uva ursi every two hours until symptoms improve. The dosage will depend on whether it is a tea, capsule, or tincture.

☞ If citrus fruits aggravate your bladder, avoid them.

☞ Prevention suggestions include drinking liquids frequently and urinating as soon as possible after you feel the urge and after sex.

JOINT DISORDERS

Back Pain

Pain in the back may be caused by a strain or sprain, by misalignment of the spinal vertebrae, or by pelvic bones causing pressure on neves. Back tension and spasms may also be caused by emotional states such as anger or fear.

Symptoms

Pain is present in the affected part of the back. The low back and neck are the most common sites of acute back pain. It is sometimes difficult and painful for the person to move or straighten up. Pain may be either dull or quite sharp, particularly when moving about. Muscles around the site of the pain are often in spasm.

Complications

Some acute back pain may be caused by a herniated vertebral disk. This type of pain usually extends into a limb and may be quite severe and accompanied by numbness. It is usually worse when sneezing, coughing or holding the breath, and bearing down. Acute pain in the mid-back may be caused by kidney stones or a kidney infection. Medical attention should be sought immediately for proper diagnosis, especially if fever is present or the pain is excruciating.

Homoeopathic Medicines

☞ Give Arnica for sore, bruised back pain after an injury or trauma.

☞ Arnica is used before and after back surgery to promote healing.

☞ Bryonia is the best medicine when the main symptom is pain that is made worse by moving.

☞ Hypericum is good for direct injuries to the spine or neves, with shooting pain.

☞ Give Rhus toxicodendron when the pain is made worse by overexertion and getting wet, and better by limbering up and moving around.

Self Care and Home Remedies

☞ When the injury first occurs, apply an ice pack if there is swelling or inflammation.

☞ After twelve to twenty four hours, apply moist heat to the area.

☞ Take a hot bath with one cup of Epsom salts added. Whirlpool baths or hot tubs are also good.

☞ Rest in bed is a comfortable position.

☞ Acupuncture, chiropractic, osteopathy, physical therapy, Bowen therapy (an Australian bodywork technique), massage, or other bodywork techniques are often helpful if homoeopathy is not producing immediate results.

SPRAINS AND STRAINS

A sprain is an injury to the muscles, tendons, and ligaments—the connective tissues that surround joints. Sprains and strains results from twisting, turning, moving, of falling in such a way as to cause an injury. They can also result from overuse.

Symptoms

Pain (mild to severe) and stiffness are the main symptoms of sprains and strains.

Complications

In cases of severe pain, it is helpful to seek immediate attention and, if appropriate, obtain an X-ray to make sure there are no fractures or dislocations.

Homoeopathic Medicines

☞ The best medicine to give first for sprains and strains is Arnica.

☞ If the pain is worse from any motion, give Bryonia.

☞ If the injured area is cold to the touch and the pain is better from cold applications, Ledum is the best medicine.

☞ If the main symptom is stiffness that is better from moving around and stretching, Rhus toxicodendron will be of benefit.

☞ If there is injury to ligaments or tendons without any clear picture that points to one of the other medicines, give Ruta.

Self Care and Home Remedies

☞ Ice the injured area. Sports medicine doctors used to recommend icing for the first twenty-four to forty-eight hours, then applying heat, but now many suggest continuing to apply ice to the injury. Icing reduces swelling and inflammation.

☞ Rest the injured area. If necessary immobilise it, including using crutches.

☞ Wrap the injured part with an elastic bandage.

☞ Apply an ointment, cream, or gel of topical Arnica.

☞ Soak in an Epsom salt tub or foot bath to help reduce swelling.

SCIATICA

Sciatica is pain along the distribution of the sciatic nerve in the back of the leg, resulting from inflammation and compression of the nerve at its root near the spine, in the buttocks, or in the pelvis. The nerve compression in the spine often comes from a herniated intervertebral disk.

Symptoms

Pain begins in the back or pelvis and radiates down the leg partially or all the way to the foot. The pain may be quite severe and accompanied by numbness and tingling. It is usually worse when sneezing, coughing, or holding the breath and bearing down.

Complications

The disk problem can get worse if lifting and straining are not done properly, increasing the sciatic pain sometimes to the point of incapacitation.

Homoeopathic Medicines

☞ If there are lots of twitching and spasms in a person who seems intoxicated, think of Agaricus.

☞ If the sciatica comes on after anger or being offended, give Colocynthis.

☞ If the sciatica is on the right side and has pain along with numbness, give Gnaphhalium.

☞ If the sciatica is from an injury to the spine, Hypericum is probably the right medicine.

☞ If the person wakes in the early morning with the sciatica, give Kali iodatum.

☞ If other symptoms are left sided, but the sciatica is right sided, think of Lachesis.

☞ If the symptoms are worse from sitting and better from moving around, consider Rhus toxicodendron.

☞ If a herniated disk is definitely involved consider Tellurium, especially if the person also has ringworm.

Self Care and Home Remedies

☞ Apply moist heat to the low back and buttocks.

☞ Take a hot bath with one cup of Epsom salts added.

☞ Rest in bed in a comfortable position.

☞ Acupuncture, chiropractic, osteopathy, physical therapy, or massage may be helpful if homoeopathy is not producing immediate results.

☞ Take Calcium (1500 mg) and Magnesium (750 mg) daily to reduce muscle spasms.

☞ Arnica gel or oil is very helpful when applied locally to the area.

8

Ayurvedic Cure of Disorders of Kidney and Urinary System

BURNING (SENSATION DURING URINATION)

- Powder equal quantities of liquorice (mulathi) and cumin (jeera). Take 1/4 teaspoon everyday along with 1 teaspoon honey for a month.
- Grind 2 to 3 teaspoons dried pomegranate seeds (annar daana) and take once or twice along with milk.
- Add 1 to 2 drops of sandalwood oil to milk and take as a night cap at bedtime.

Urination Scanty

- Boil 1/4 teaspoon powdered green cardamom (chhoti illaichi) seeds in thin tea water and drink.

Urine Retention

- Soak a little saffron (kesar) overnight in one cup of water. Next morning drink it with 1 teaspoon honey.

Bladder Stones

- Boil 2 figs (anjeer) in 1 cup of water. Drink daily for a month.
- For any sort of this trouble, soak about 5 to 7 gms. of tulsi seeds in water, add a little of sugar to the combination to make it more tasty. Drink this combination early in the morning and also in the afternoon, i.e. twice a day. Soon you will have copious discharge of urine and all problems connected with the urinary tract shall vanish in a week's time. Continue drinking raw milk and water mixture at least twice a day also.

Kidney Malfunctioning

- Frequent intake of coriander (dhania) tea: boil or steep 2 teaspoons coriander (dhania) powder in a glass of boiling hot water. Add sugar and milk to taste.
- Add more almonds to the daily diet.

Stones in the Gall Bladder

- Hot fomentation on the back as well as lower abdomen is always useful for relieving pain.
- To treat this problem first boil the pieces of beetroot in water and crush the pieces in this water fully. When cool, strain the potion and drink this water every morning, afternoon and evening. In about a week's time the stones will melt and pass out with urine.

Bed Wetting in Children

- Give 2 walnut halves (akhrot giri) and 1 teaspoon of kishmish to the child before sleeping for 10-12 days.

Painful Urination

- Carrot juice is a diuretic substance. If you have any problem connected with urination, have a glass of carrot juice every morning and evening. This will make the sufferer urinate frequently and all the problems connected with urine shall vanish. Even otherwise, drinking carrot juice would help keep the urinary tract clean and unobstructed.
- Mix 1/2 teaspoon powdered fenugreek seeds (methi daana) in buttermilk and drink.
- Add 1 tablespoon mint (pudina) leaves to 1 cup water. Take twice or thrice a day.
- Take 5 drops of sandalwood oil along with 1 cup of milk. Add a pinch of powdered carom seeds (ajwain), drink it.

Ayurvedic Cure of Disorders of Muscles and Joints

In our daily life, we suffer from sprain, backache and bodyaches. Here are the remedies for various muscular and joint disorders.

Sprain

- Chop raw onions and put in a towel. Place this over the sprain to relieve pain and bring down the swelling. Alternatively, make a footbath of lavender oil and water and soak your ankle, but do not massage the area.
- Grind lime leaves into a fine paste. Mix it with an equal quantity of butter. Apply on the affected areas.
- Mix equal parts of almonds oil & garlic oil and massage over the affected parts.
- Take 1 gram flour, just a pinchful of salt, and add half of its quantity with equal amount of turmeric powder. Add linseed oil in it or any other oil like of mustard or til, and make the poultice. Apply it on the sprained portion. The poultice will enhance the blood circulation and in two days' time the relief will be there.

Muscular Cramps

- Apply clove oil on the affected parts.

Muscular Pain

- Warm the papaya leaf over the fire and apply on affected parts.

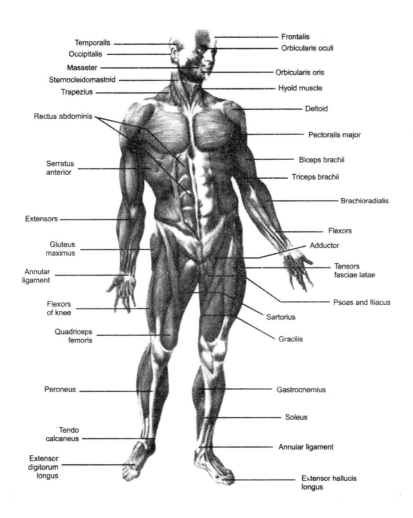

- Heat ginger (adrak) paste with turmeric (haldi) paste (1:1) and apply.
- Soak ½ teaspoon liquoric (mulathi) root powder in 1 cup water and leave overnight. Mix into the infusion 1 cup rice gruel (cooked broken rice) and take every morning.

Rib Pain

- Grind a turmeric piece and mix in a hot water to form a thick paste. Apply this paste over the ribs aching. Soon the pain will vanish. In case you feel you are not having the desired effect, prepare the oil of turmeric and lightly massage your aching ribs with this oil. Another treatment for quick relief is to mix turmeric powder in the milk of the Aak plant (the medicinal plant, swallow wort, whose botanical name is Calotropes Gigantea) and apply over the ribs. This paste will quickly give relief.

Ankle Swelling and Pain

- Mix equal quantities of castor oil and lime juice. Massage the affected area with the mixture. Also drink 1 cup warm water mixed with lime juice and honey.

Heels Having Pain

- Mix equal amounts by weight of carom seeds (ajwain) onion seeds (kalaunji), fenugreek seeds (methi daana) and saboot isabgol. Have 1 tablespoon everyday first thing in the morning. If you can grind them slightly in the mixer—makes it more effective. This treatment takes a couple of months but is a sure shot remedy.

Note: Saboot isabgol, tiny very light pinkish particles, will be available with your grocer or if you request him he will get it for you from the wholesale market. Do not use the husk which is generally used by people for constipation as that is less effective but not harmful. If saboot isabgol is not available, husk can be used. It takes longer for the pain to go.

Legs, Swelling and Pain

- Mix equal quantities of castor oil and lime juice. Massage the affected area with this mixture. Also drink 1 cup warm water mixed with lime juice and honey.

Athletes's Foot

Keeping your feet clean and dry is enough to discourage the growth of this fungal infection. Remember, it is infectious and you must keep and wash your shoes, socks, and towel separately. To sooth the broken areas of your feet, simply soak them for 10 minutes in a foot-both of apple cider vinegar mixed with water.

Foot Corns

- Tie a fresh slice of lemon over the corn (painful area) and keep it all night.
- Massage castor oil on the corns every morning and night before sleeping.
- Massage for 2-3 minutes so that the oil gets absorbed. In 3-4 weeks the corns will disappear.
- Mash 1-2 cloves (laung) & garlic (lahasun) and tie over the corns. Keep overnight.

Sciatica

- Take just 10 gms. of turmeric and grind it in 100 gms. of cow's urine. Add about 25 gms. of castor oil to it and make the patient drink the whole lot. The patient will get relief. Alternatively make the patient inhale deeply the vapours emerging out of the large vessel in which jaggery is being prepared from the sugar cane juice. But the patient must keep his body covered with a heavy blanket. The more he sweats, the quicker he will be cured.

Paralysis

- Boil a few leaves of tulsi in a tumblerful of water. When cool, strain and put this water in a bottle. Massage this water on the affected limbs. Continue this treatment for at least two weeks. This treatment, coupled with regular intake of the tulsi leaves as an alternative treatment along with other remedies is helpful in giving good results.

Fainting

- A hot poultice of carom seeds (ajwain) may be used as dry fomentation for hands and feet.

Gout-Swelling

- Take 250 gms. of turmeric powder, 50 gms; Kuchala powder, 50 gms; pigeon dung, 100 gms; castor oil and 250 gms. til oil. Mix both the oils, add turmeric, kuchala and pigeons dung and boil. When the solid contents turn black, coot and strain the oil mixture. Add to it a cup of kerosene oil. Repeatedly massage this oil on your joints. Always massage the adjoining areas before massaging the swollen part. Like if you have to massage your knees, first massage the upper thigh and thigh joint before massaging the knees. This way the raw phlegm will be dissolved and not shifted to other portion. Try not to have constipation when you take this massage course.

Gouty Pains

- Mix mustard oil and rectified alcohol (1 part oil to 40 parts alcohol) and use as a lotion.
- Make a poultice of ground fenugreek seeds (methi dana) use on the affected part.
- Equal quantities of Asparagus seeds (halong). Black cumin, fenugreek (methi) and ajwain should be taken and swallowed every morning in dose of 3 grams. The remedies are also recommended for rheumatism and lumbago.

Rheumatism

- Heat the leaves of the plant swallow wort (Aak in Hindi) and tie them over the affected joints.

- Grind the guava leaves to a paste form and apply on the affected joint.
- Take about 750 gms. of the root of Arand plant and boil it in 6 kgs. of water. When it is reduced to $1/4^{th}$ of its normal quantity, then add castor oil to it and boil again till whole of the water in the mixture evaporates leaving only the oily substance. Strain this oil through a fine muslin cloth and keep it preserved, in a glass bottle. Massage your limbs with this oil at least 15 mts. before you go to have your bath. In case you do it after your bath, then tie cotton wads after the massage over the affected joints.
- Take 'Binaules', cut, grind and sieve them and boil in water, when only thick paste remains. Dry it and then tie it over your affected joints.

Rheumatic Pain

- Boil 3 tablespoon powdered nutmeg (jaiphal) in 1 cup of sesame oil (til ka tel). Cool and apply on affected parts.
- 2 to 3 teaspoon pepper powder is fried in 2 teaspoons of sesame oil (til ka tel) until charred. When it is warm, it is applied on the affected areas and massaged lightly.
- A 3 inch piece of dried ginger is grinded with a grape sized piece of asafoetida (hing) in milk. The paste is applied on the affected area. The area is exposed to the sun for imparting warmth and heat.
- The patient must avoid fried eatables and sour foods like curds and alcohol, moong dal, meat soup, garlic, onions, bitter gourd, papaya and green bananas are the foods which help in controlling gout and rheumatic pain.

Joint Pain

- Take equal quantities of asparagus seeds (shatavari), black cumin seeds (shah jeera), fenugreek (methi

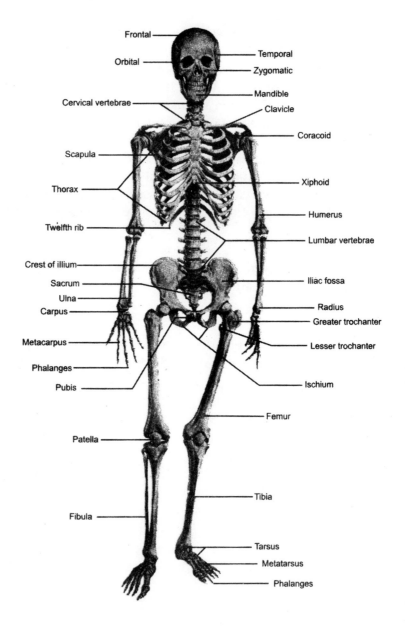

daana) seeds and carom seeds (ajwain). Powder and take 1/2 teaspoon every morning.

- Combine 6 teaspoons each of ginger (adrak) and caraway seeds along with 3 teaspoons of black pepper corns (saboot kali mirch) and grind into a fine powder. Have ½ teaspoon with water twice daily.
- Soak 1-2 teaspoons fenugreek seeds (methi daana) in a cup of curd overnight. Eat in the morning on an empty stomach or soak 1-2 teaspoons fenugreek seeds (methi daana) in 1 cup water overnight. Drink the water first thing in the morning and also eat the methi seeds.
- Take out 1 tablespoon juice of fresh leaves of bathua and drink every day on an empty stomach for 2-3 months. Do not add anything to the juice and do not eat anything before and after, for 2 hours.
- Make a tea from papaya seeds and have 6-7 cups a day, for at least 2 weeks.
- Have 1-2 garlic (lahasun) cloves or 1 garlic, which has only 1 clove in a pod, first thing in the morning.
- Mix 1 teaspoon of dry amla powder with 2 teaspoons of jaggery (gur) and have it twice daily for a month.

Arthritis

Extract the juice of carrots and add to it the juice of Karnphool (Dandelion). Have just 5 gms. of carrot juice and add only half of the quantity the juice of dandelion. Drink this combination regularly for at least 15 days for speedier relief. It is also advisable to rub Mahanarayani oil on the joints.

Bed Sores

- Apply honey on the length and breadth of a banana leave and lie on it for a few hours. Ensure its contact with the affected parts.

Body Pain

- Boil 3 tablespoons powdered nutmeg (jaiphal) in 1 cup of sesame oil (til ka tel), coot it and apply on affected parts.

Body Swelling

- Grind black cumin seeds (shah jeera) with a little hot water and apply on affected parts.

Body and Muscles Development

- Soak 2 almonds, 5 pista kernels and 1 teaspoon poppy seeds in 1 cup cow's milk for an hour. Grind it and add some more warm milk. Take daily for 3 months.

Bruises

- Slice a raw onion and place over the bruises. Do not apply this to broken skin.

Fatigue

- Take a glass of grapefruit and lemon juice in equal parts to dispel fatigue and general tiredness after a days' work.

Body Weakness

- Soak 8 to 10 almonds and 1 teaspoon rice overnight. Remove the outer skin of almonds. Grind into a fine paste. Mix in some milk and pinch of turmeric powder (haldi). Boil and drink along with sugar candy (mishri) or ordinary sugar to taste.
- Sprinkle the following on a platter of mango slices; 1 teaspoon honey, a pinch of saffron (kesar), cardamom (chhoti illaichi) and rose water (gulab jal). Take twice daily.

Exhaustion due to Overwork

- Boil ¼ teaspoon powdered cardamom (chhoti illaichi) seeds in thin tea water and drink.

(10)

Skin Disorders

Skin is the outer covering of our body which protects us from several infectious agents.

ALLERGIC REACTIONS

Allergic reactions can be mild or severe. They occur when the body is exposed to an allergen—a substance in the environment that causes an immune-system response. The response is triggered by the release of histamine from the mast cells, which are part of the immune system. Allergic reactions are caused by an immune-system response that is greater than is needed to respond to the presence of a foreign substance in the body.

Symptoms

Allergic symptoms include swelling, itching, redness, inflammation, sneezing, mucous discharges, hives or other skin rashes, asthma, and systemic shock, as seen in an anaphylactic response.

Complications

Anaphylactic shock and respiratory arrest: If the person has a severe reaction to an allergen, including significant itching and swelling of lymph nodes, swelling of the mucous membranes of the nose and ears, and difficult breathing due to constriction of the air passages, this is likely to be an anaphylactic response and requires emergency care. If untreated, anaphylaxis can be rapidly fatal.

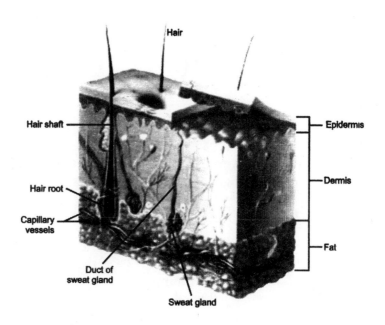

Homoeopathic Medicines

☞ If the person's nose runs like a faucer with streaming eyes, think of Allium cepa.

☞ If swelling and stinging pains are the most prominent symptoms, consider Apis.

☞ If anxiety and restlessness are the most significant symptoms, think of Arsenicum.

☞ If symptoms occur after getting wet or over work, and stiffness and itching eruptions are present, give Rhustox.

☞ If the allergic reaction is to shellfish, or feels like stinging nettles or a burn, give Urtica urens.

Self Care and Home Remedies

☞ For shock: lie down, keep warm, drink fluids.

☞ For itching: Soak in a bathtub of warm water with one cup of baking soda or one cup of raw oatmeal.

☞ For swelling: ice pack or cold wet compresses.

Frostbite

Frostbite is the freezing of a part of the body from exposure to cold.

Symptoms

The affected body part becomes cold, hard, and white as it is actually frozen, and is usually not painful until it warms up again. The part may become red, itching and throbbing on rewarming, and blistering may occur.

Complications

If severe, frostbite may lead to gangrene, in which the tissue becomes black and eventually sloughs off. The limb may require amputation as a result of the gangrene. If the frostbitten area is black, seek medical attention immediately.

Homoeopathic Medicines

☞ Agaricus is always the first medicine to consider for frostbite.

☞ In mild frostbite with splinter like pains, Nitric acid is the best choice.

☞ If there is bluish red discoloration, itching, and pain, especially in the feet, consider Pulsatilla.

☞ If the frostbitten area feels worse from rubbing and the person has restless legs, give Zincum metallicum.

Self Care and Home Remedies

☞ Do not apply ice or snow to the frozen part.

☞ Rewarm the part as soon as possible, preferably with circulating warm water or contact with warmth, but not with excessive heat.

HIVES

Hives appear on the skin as part of an allergic reaction to a food or an environmental allergen such as pollen, dust mites or wool. Hives may also occur due to exercise or from becoming cold.

Symptoms

Hives are red, raised welts that are often quite itchy, hot, and swollen.

Complications

In a serious case of acute hives, anaphylaxis (characterised by intense itching, swelling, and difficulty in breathing due to constriction of the bronchioles) can be life—threatening and requires emergency medical attention. Hives may become chronic or may occur repeatedly if the allergen that causes the body to react is not eliminated.

Homoeopathic Medicines

☞ If there is tremendous swelling, give Apis first.

☞ For hives due to bee stings, give Apis.

☞ If itching is the main symptom and the person is very restless, give Rhus toxicodendron.

☞ If the hives sting and there is not significant swelling, consider Urtica urens.

Self Care and Home Remedies

☞ For itching: Soak in a bathtub of warm water with one cup of baking soda or one cup of raw oatmeal.

☞ For swelling: Ice pack or cold wet compresses.

☞ Take 500 mg Vitamin C twice a day.

Cold Sores

Cold sores are caused by a virus, Herpes Simplex Virus I, which remains dormant in the nerve roots around the mouth. Episodes of outbreaks occur whenever stress levels are too high and the immune system is not strong enough to keep the virus in check. Exposure to the sun can also cause a recurrence.

symptoms

Single or multiple blisters, which may be as large as a dime, usually occur cn or around the lips. The blisters are often accompanied by swelling and are usually quite painful. Numbness and tingling may occur before the blisters appear, as well as fatigue.

Complications

Cold sores will usually disappear on their own in one to two weeks. There are usually no complications, although scarring may occur in some cases.

Homoeopathic Medicines

☞ Natrum muriaticum is the most frequently used medicine for cold sores.

☞ For cold sores that come on from exposure to the sun in a sensitive person who easily gets her feelings hurt, the most common medicine is Natrum muriaticum.

☞ Cold sores that burn in a chilly, anxious, restless person may require Arsenicum album.

☞ People needing Hepar sulphuris are generally extremely chilly and their sensitivity to the pain of the cold sores seems out of proportion.

☞ Cold sores that occur after exertion or exposure to cold, damp weather usually respond to Rhus toxicodendron.

Self Care and Home Remedies

☞ Lysine: 500 mg three times a day.

☞ vitamin C: 1000 mg three times a day.

☞ Beta carotene: 50,000 IU a day.

☞ Zinc: 30 mg a day.

☞ One part Calendula tincture mixed with three parts water applied with a cotton swab three times a day.

CONTACT DERMATITIS

Poison ivy, oak, and sumag cause a contact dermatitis. Some people are highly sensitive to these plants, and some show no sensitivity. Poison ivy and sumac are more common in the eastern part of the United States, and poison oak in the west. The oil of these plants can be spread around the body by touch. It can also cause a severe reaction if the plants are burned and the smoke inhaled.

Symptoms

An extremely itchy, red, blistering rash that causes great discomfort and annoyance, and often takes more than a week to heal. The blisters ooze and crust over before drying up.

Complications

These skin rashes are usually self limiting and cause no long term effects. The homeopathic proving of poison ivy suggests that arthritis could be a long term complication if the skin rash is suppressed by external applications such as hydro-cortisone cream.

Homoeopathic Medicines

- ☞ Anacardium is often the most effective medicine for poison ivy, oak, and sumac.
- ☞ Croton tiglium can be used if the skin feels incredibly itchy and hidebound, and there is gushing diarrhea.
- ☞ Rhus toxicodendron is the most available medicine, and will often work.

Self Care and Home Remedies

- ☞ Be careful not to spread the rash by scratching it, then scratching an unaffected area.
- ☞ Wash the area with mild soap and water and cover with sterile gauze, if needed, to keep it clean.
- ☞ Calendula lotion is soothing to the rash and irritated skin.
- ☞ Cold wet applications can help the rash feel better, especially cold comfrey root tea.

☞ Oatmeal bath: Use Aveno or place one cup of finely blended dry Oatmeal in the bath to sooth itching.

☞ If secondary infection from scratching occurs, cleanse with Calendula soap and water and apply Calendula gel or lotion.

SKIN INFECTIONS: BOILS, FOLLICULITIS AND CARBUNCLES

Boils, folliculitis, and carbuncles are skin infections, usually associated with Staphylococcus aureus bacteria.

Symptoms

Folliculitis is an infection of the hair follicules with redness, tenderness, and swelling. Boils, also called furuncles, are more advanced skin infections which form a large eruption that discharges bloody pus. Boils are most common on the neck, face, breasts, and buttocks. Boils can be quite painful and especially tender to pressure. A collection of boils that forms one large infected area penetrating deeper into the tissue is called a carbuncle. Carbuncles are common at the base of the neck. They may be accompanied by fatigue and fever. They are slow to heal, slough off tissue with blood and pus, and can cause scarring.

Complications

Skin infections can lead to a serious systemic blood infection called septicemia. The symptoms of septicemia are a high fever and organ damage. Septicemia can be fatal. Red streaks extending from the infected area toward the heart are a red flag for septicemia and indicate a need for immediate medical attention.

Homoeopathic Medicines

☞ For crusty, oozing, black eruptions, give Anthracinum.

☞ For infections with small, red, ulcerated pimples and burning pains, consider Arsenicum album, especially if the person is nervous and restless.

☞ If the person screams when you examine the infected area, give Hepar sulphuris.

☞ If the infected area is bluish purple and left- sided, consider Lachesis.

☞ For infections with bad smelling discharges and perspiration and bad breath, Mercurius is the first thought.

☞ For infections due to an ingrown nail, think first of Silica.

Self Care and Home Remedies

☞ Hot, moist packs can be helpful for folliculitis and boils to bring the infection to a head.

☞ An echinacea and goldenseal combination (two drop-perfuls of tincture in water three times a day or six capsules a day) is useful to stimulate the immune system to fight infection.

☞ Give Vitamin A (25,000 IU a day) or beta carotene (50,000 IU a day).

☞ Give Vitamin C (1000 mg three times a day).

☞ Give Zinc (30 mg a day).

DIAPER RASH

Diaper rash is a skin irritation or infection which occurs when wet diapers stay in prolonged contact with the baby's skin.

Symptoms

The skin is moist, red and raw. Red spots or patches may indicate a yeast infection due to Candida. Bacterial infection may cause blistering and pus.

Complications

Diaper rash rarely causes anything other than local inflammation or infection. If a high fever is present without another obvious cause and the lymph glands in the groin are swollen, seek medical attention to rule out an infection in the blood stream.

Homoeopathic Medicines

☞ Babies needing Hepar sulphuris are generally extremely chilly and very sensitive to uncovering. They have an infected diaper rash with pus that smells like rotten cheese.

☞ Infants who need Graphites have diaper rash in the folds of the skin, which is dry, red, cracked, and very itchy, with a honey like discharge that crusts over.

☞ Babies needing medorrhinum have a sharply demarcated red, sometimes shiny diaper rash often caused by Candida infection, called "thrush diaper rash."

☞ Infants who need Sulphur have a red, dry, itchy diaper rash around the anus that is worse from getting overheated and from a warm bath.

Self Care and Home Remedies

☞ Let the baby go without diapers whenever possible.

☞ Change diapers whenever they become wet or soiled.

☞ Cleanse the area with very mild soap and water.

☞ Dry the area carefully with a hairdryer on the lowest heat.

☞ Apply Calendula cream after every diaper change until diaper rash is gone.

☞ Cornstarch may be useful on the skin as a drying powder.

☞ Use all cotton diapers instead of rubber pants.

11

Ayurvedic Cure of Skin and Hair Problems

ACNE

- Pound a piece of radish to a pulp and just apply this pulp on the face. Keep is till it is dry. Then rub it off by cold water. Internally, consume radish, its juice and the radish vegetable cooked by steam heat. It is better to leave salt altogether till your blood is clean. The acne results because of impurity of blood.
- Mix 1 teaspoon lemon juice in 1 teaspoon finely grind cinnamon (dalchini) powder and apply on affected areas frequently. Sift the cinnamon (dalchini) powder to make it into a very fine powder.
- Crush a few garlic (lahasun) flakes and apply on the face, once or twice a day. Swallowing 1-2 flakes of raw garlic regularly helps further.
- Grind some neem leaves with water to a fine paste. Apply on infected area.
- Make a paste of 1/2 teaspoon each of sandalwood and turmeric (haldi) powder in little water and apply.
- Grind some black cumin seeds (Jeera) with a little vinegar (sirka) to a smooth paste. Apply on affected parts.
- Clean face with cotton wool dipped in rose water 2-3 times a day. Do not use soap.
- Orange peel is very good in the treatment of acne. Grind the peel with some water to a paste and apply on affected parts. When oranges are not in season, you

may use a powder of dried orange peels. For this, when oranges are in season, dry orange peels in shade. Powder finely in a grinder and sift it to make it a very fine powder. Store in an air tight bottle for future use.

Blackheads

- Mix 1 teaspoon lime juice in 1 teaspoon finely grind cinnamon (dalchini) powder and apply on affected areas frequently.
- Mix 1 teaspoon each turmeric (haldi) powder and juice of fresh coriander (dhania) leaves and apply daily as a face before going to sleep.

Pimples

- Grind equal quantity of nutmeg (jaiphal), black pepper (kali mirch) and sandalwood. Apply on affected area.
- Clean face with rose water (gulab) 2-3 times a day.
- The orange peel (santre ka chilka) is very valuable in the treatment of acne and pimples. Pound the peel with water on a piece of stone and apply on the affected area. When oranges are not in season, dry peels in the shade. Powder the dried peels. Sift to get a fine powder and store.
- Rub nutmeg (jaiphal) in unboiled milk to form a paste. Apply on the face and let it dry. Wash it off with warm water. Do it 2-3 times a day. You will see the pimples disappearing in 3-4 days.
- A couple of garlic (lahasun) cloves crushed and rubbed on the face 1-2 times a day. This process is further helped by taking raw garlic regularly. Have 1-2 cloves in the morning.
- Apply fresh lemon juice on the affected area overnight. Wash off with warm water next morning.
- Grind some neem leaves with water to a fine paste. Apply on infected area.

- Application of fresh mint (pudina) juice over face every night cures pimples and prevents dryness of the skin.
- Mix equal amounts of lemon juice and rose water (gulab jal). Apply on face and keep for ½ an hour. 15-20 days of this application helps cure pimples and also removes blemishes and scars.

Scars on Face

- Wash face with coconut water (nariyal pani). Apply coconut water on face and leave for 15-20 minutes before washing it off.
- Grind one teaspoon yellow mustard (peeli rai) to a paste with 1 tablespoon malai/cream and apply on face and neck. Leave for 15-20 minutes. This also removes itching as well as blemishes from the skin.
- Wash and grind a few fresh mint (pudina) leaves to a smooth paste. Apply and leave for 1/2 an hour or apply every night before going to sleep. This helps in getting rid of pimples along with the blemishes.
- Apply a teaspoon of olive oil mixed with 1/2 teaspoon of lime juice, leave it for 20-25 minutes and then wash off.
- Take the pulp of a ripe tomato. Add a few drops of lemon juice and rub on the face and neck. Leave for 20-25 minutes before washing.
- If your skin is dry, rub a stick of sandalwood in milk and if skin is oily, rub it in rose water (gulab jal) and then apply on face. Leave for an hour and then wash with cold water. This is very effective during summers.
- For a dry & blemished skin, mix a tablespoon gram flour (besan), add a pinch of turmeric (haldi), 1/4 teaspoon orange peel (or santre ka chilka) powder, a teaspoon curd (dahi) and a teaspoon of milk. Apply on face and neck. When skin feels taunt, rub it off with finger tips, and wash off with tap water.

Scars Due to Burn

- Boil 1 cup neem bark in 4 cups water. Remove from fire and shake liquid. Apply the emerging froth on the affected area. Repeat several times and for several days.
- Blanch and grind a few almonds to a fine paste with 2 tablespoons milk and one tablespoon each of orange and carrot juice. Apply well on the face and neck. Leave for 1/2 an hour, then wash off.
- Apply one tablespoon finely grind raw papaya on face and neck. Keep for 15-20 minutes and wash off.

Pustules

- Take half kg turmeric powder and boil it and add about 200 gms. of pure honey to it. Keep the mixture as it is for two weeks in a glass jar. Now strain it and fill in a clean bottle. Take 10 to 15 gms. of this Aasav (mixture) after food. This will cleanse your blood of the impurities which cause pustules. Also dip a cotton piece in turmeric oil and place it over pustules for relief.

To Open Shrinked Pores of the Skin

- Mix one tablespoon tomato juice and a few drops of lemon juice. Apply on open pores. Wash after 15-20 minutes.
- Rub a cube of ice everyday, on the area where open pores are present. Wash face with cold water. Never use hot water on face.

Face—Freckles (Jhanyin)

- These are mainly caused by using creams and lotions indiscriminately which burn the outer layer of the skin. Take just 10 gms. of grind turmeric and drench it in the milk of the banyan, peepal or aak tree. Make a thick and uniform paste of it in the evening and cover it with a lid. Keep it as it is overnight. Massag your face with this ubtan at least half an hour before you take your bath. Continue this treatment for a week to remove all the freckles. Then use ubtan just once a week.

Skin Cracked

- For dry, cracked hands apply a mixture of grated potato soaked in olive oil. Leave this on for 10 minutes and then rinse off.

The Decoction or Karha

- Decoction made out of chukander or beetroot leaves is very effective to cure this trouble. You can prepare the karha in the following manner:
- Take a few pieces of beetroot (chukander) and dice them to small pieces. Boil them in water when they become tender, crush them as much as to reduce them to a pulp. Again add a little water and boil the whole lot once again. When you find the solution becoming homogeneous and thick, cool it and strain it through a coarse cloth or strainer. The karha is ready. Wash your hands and feet with this karha everyday when you retire for the day. It is always better to keep your hands and feet immersed in this diluted karha before washing them with the water. In about a couple of days your skin will become soft and glowing. This karha would be used for application on the dry face.

Skin Allergies

- Grind 1 tablespoon poppy seeds (khuskhus) with 1 teaspoon water. Add 1 teaspoon lime juice. Apply on the affected areas.
- Mix 1 teaspoon lime juice with sandalwood paste and apply all over.

Skin Irritation

- Take clean water and rub vigorously a piece of cucumber to make its thick paste. Then apply the paste on the skin for its cure in two three days time. But the patient should not consume heat producing items like spicy food, tea and even lots of common salt.

Itching

- Extract juice of tulsi and massage on the parts of the body itching. If the trouble be chronic, take about 2 parts of tulsi juice and one part of til oil. Allow them to boil on slow fire. Then cool it and put it in a bottle. This is most effective oil for all sorts of itching problems.

Ring Worms

- Take a large piece of pure turmeric and gently rub it over a stone slab (sil) drenched with water. Take out the rubbed portion of turmeric from the stone slab and apply the paste over the rings on your body. When the paste dries apply another layer of the turmeric paste over it. In a couple of days time the trouble will start to end and the sprouts will also disappear. Don't discontinue the treatment once you get well. It is better to apply the paste for a week more for total relief.

Eczema

- Add 1 teaspoon camphor (kapoor) to 1 teaspoon sandalwood paste and apply on the affected areas.
- Mix a paste of turmeric (haldi) and neem leaves (1:1) in a little gingelly oil (til ka tel) and apply on affected areas.
- Grind 1 tablespoon each turmeric (haldi), neem leaves and gingelly oil (til ka tel) into a fine paste and apply on the affected parts.

- Rub a nutmeg (jaiphal) against a smooth stone slab with a little water and make a paste. Apply on affected parts.
- Stop using any soap and wash your body with neem soap.
- Grind pure sulphur and add in pure mustard oil and apply on your body.
- Take about 6 gms. of soda bicarb and pour in the juice of half a lemon over it. Add about 20 gms. of mustard oil and massage your body vigorously with this mixture. Then take sun-bath for about 2 hours before you go to take your bath. It is especially effective if your skin is dry.
- Extract the juice of leaves of beetroot and mixing it with honey, Apply it over the affected part. In about a week's time this trouble will end.
- Apply freshly pounded radish pulp over the affected part. Allow it to dry. In about half an hour take bath in hot water in which some perfume is added. In about a week's treatment the affliction shall be removed.

Warts

- Mash the garlic (lahasun) cloves and apply externally.
- Apply the milky juice exuding from the stems of figs (anjeer) and leaves on the affected areas.
- Place some chopped onions in a dish. Cover with salt and leave overnight. Twice a day apply the resulting juice to the warts until they disappear.
- Another alternative is fresh pineapple juice or slices. Since pineapple contains an enzyme that breaks down warts, it is very effective in removing warts without leaving behind any marks. Apply some to the warts several times in a day until it has gone.

Sunburn

- Mix 2 teaspoons tomato juice and 4 tablespoons buttermilk (chhach). Apply it. Wash after 1/2 an hour.
- Mix olive oil with equal quantity of vinegar and apply an hour before your bath.

Sweating Excessive

- Mix dry sandalwood powder in rose water (gulab jal) (1:1) and apply over parts where seating is excessive.

Thorn

- If a thorn has gone in your child's foot and is not coming out, simply mix jaggery (gur) and carom seeds (ajwain) and tie on it. The thorn will come out on it's own.

Wrinkles

- Apply coconut oil on the portions of skin and face where wrinkles set in and gently massage every night at bed time.
- Soak shhredded ginger (adrak) in honey. Eat a spoonful every morning.

Body Dry Itch

- Grind 1 tablespoon poppy seeds (khuskhus) with 1 teaspoon water. Add 1 teaspoon lime juice. Apply on the affected areas.

Body Heat

- Add 2 to 3 drops of almond oil to pomegranate (anaar) juice and drink.
- Remove seeds from fresh amla fruits and grind the pulp into a fine paste. Tie it in a muslin cloth and squeeze out the juice. Take 2 teaspoons of this juice and mix it with two teaspoonfuls each honey and lime juice.

Add 1 cup water and drink on an empty stomach every morning.

- Take a tender bel fruit. Grind it with 1 cup milk. Apply on the head and massage well before taking a shower.
- Soak 8 to 10 almonds and 1 teaspoon rice overnight. Remove the outer skin. Grind into a fine paste. Mix with some milk and add a pinch of turmeric powder (haldi) and sugar candy (mishri) to taste. Boil and drink.

Burns by Fire

- Immediately apply glycerine on the burnt area.
- Burn a handful of mango leaves to ashes and apply this on the affected parts.

Burns by Hot Water

- Take the thin bugs of banana leaves. Bandage directly on affected areas. Tie the upper part for two days and then lower parts for two more days.

Palms, Burning Sensation

- Grind a handful of bitter gourd (karela) leaves into a smooth paste and apply on the affected areas of feet and palms frequently.
- Finely grind a handful of henna (mehendi) leaves and add 2 tablespoon lime juice. Stir and apply on the feet.
- Apply finely grated bottle gourd (lauki) on the feet.
- Mash 1 ripe banana along with a little curd and water, take twice a day.
- Grind a handful of bitter gourd (karela) leaves into a smooth paste and apply on the affected areas of feet and palms frequently.

Heat Exhaustion

- Apply some sandalwood oil on the forehead.

Heat Stroke

- Have the cooling drink 'panna'. To prepare this, cook unripe or green mangoes in hot ashes. Extract the pulp and mix with water and sugar. You may even pressure cook the mangoes if you cannot make provision for the ashes.

Prickly Heat

- Mix dry sandalwood powder with rose water (Gulab jal) to make a paste. Apply on affected parts. When dry, wash it off. It prevents excessive sweating and heals inflammed skin.

Burns, Scar

- Boil 1 cup neem bark (neem ki khal) in 4 cups water. Remove from fire and shake liquid. Apply the emerging froth on the affected area. Repeat several times and for several days.

Burns on Body

- Apply curry leaves (kari patta) as poultices over affected areas.
- Spread a thin layer of honey over the burn and cover with a dressing. Repeat this regularly every two or three hours till it heals.
- Mash a ripe banana and apply on burns. Bandage with betel leaves (pan ka patta).
- If you have a minor burn, immediately place an ice pack on the burnt area for 10 minutes.
- Combine 4 teaspoons each of lime juice coconut oil and rub until the mixture turns white. Apply on affected parts.

Cracked Feet/Soles

- Finely grind a handful of heena (mehendi) leaves. Add 2 tablespoons lemon juice and apply on the feet.

- Mix the juice of bottle gourd (lauki) and sesame oil (til ka tel) in the ratio 4:1 and heat till the moisture has evaporated. Bottle and use over cracked skin.
- Mix equal quantities of glyceine and lemon juice. Apply every night before going to bed. This mixture can be made and stored in a glass bottle.
- Massage your feet with castor oil every night (in winters) for 2-3 minutes and then wear socks at night.
- Grind equal amounts of neem leaves and turmeric (haldi). Apply on affected area.

Feet Smelling Bad

- Soak feet in strong tea for 20 minutes everyday until the smell disappears. To prepare your footbath, dip two tea bogs in 500 ml of water for 15 minute and pour the tea into a basin containing two litres (10 cups) of cool water.

Unpleasant Body Odour

- Soak 10-15 basil leaves in 1 cup water and eat every morning for a month.
- Grind neem (azadiracta indica) leaves and apply in armpits & on other parts of body.

Black Spots

- These may be caused by excessive indulgence in the sexual pleasures which sap your vitality and these black spots appear. Extract a little juice of tulsi and add two times more lime juice. Make their homogeneous solution and apply this solution or paste over these spots every night with soft hands. The spots will be removed in a week's time.

Boils

- Slightly roast big onion on a naked flame. Mash it and mix in a teaspoon each turmeric powder and ghee. Apply and tie a bandage.

- Mash the garlic (lahasun) cloves and apply externally.
- Grind neem leaves into a paste and apply on affected parts.
- Apply a paste of ginger (adrak) powder and turmeric (haldi) 1:1) on boils.
- Grind some black cumin seeds (kala jeera) in a little water and apply the paste on the affected areas.
- Heat black pepper powder in 1/2 teaspoon ghee untill charred. Use this as an ointment.
- Take fenugreek leaf (mehi patta) paste, heat it and when lukewarm, apply on the affected part of the body.
- Soak bread in warm milk and sandwich the mixture in between the folds of a clean cotton cloth. Apply this Poultice to the boil and hold in place with a cotton bandage.This draws the dirt to the surface of the skin and simultaneously bursts the boil.

Hair Falling

- Take a handful of neem leaves and boil them in 2 cups of water. After cooling and filtering, use the decoction for rinsing hair.

Baldness

- Collect the soft and green leaves of beetroot and boil a few in water. When the leaves become tender and soft take them out of the water. Now grind the leaves fully to a homogeneous pulp. If water is needed, only that water should be used in which the leaves had been boiled.
- Repeat the procedure in a similar way but this time replacing the beetroot leaves with henna. Now grind both the leaves together. Apply this paste over the head liberally. Allow it to dry and then wash it with lukewarm water in which a few drops of lime juice have been added. Repeat the process for one full

month. It is expected that within this period hair will again start to sprout on the bald area. After doing this treatment for one full month, repeat it after every week. It is a very good remedy and many bald people have now lush growth of hair. But, as told earlier, it could be useful only when the baldness has not been due to the hereditary factor.

- Rub on the scalp 1 teaspoon oil in which raw mangoes have been preserved for over one year. Repeat this treatment frequently.
- Grind 1 tablespoon liquorice root pieces (mulathi) in 1 cup milk with 1/4 teaspoon saffron (kesar). Apply this paste on bald patches at bedtime continuously.
- Grind fenugreek seeds (methi daana), with water and apply on the head. Leave for at least 10 minutes before washing. Do it every morning for a month.
- Boil 1 cup mustard oil (sarson ka tel) with 4 tablespoon henna (mehendi) leaves. Filter and bottle. (Massage on the bald patches regularly.)
- Grind the remains of tobacco smoked in a hookah and add to boiling mustard oil. Cool and store. Massage on the bald patches regularly.

Hair Greying

- Wet a lemon half and rub lemon juice into the scalp well.Wash off after it runs dry.
- Grind 1 tablespoon each, pulp of amla and lime juice. Massage this into the hair before going to bed. Wash it next morning.
- Soak shredded ginger (adrak) in honey. Eat a spoonful every morning.

Hair Thinning

- Bathe the hair in 1 cup coconut milk twice or thrice a week for a few months.

Lice

- Grind the seeds of neem into a fine powder and mix in some groundnut oil. Apply to the scalp. Allow it to remain overnight. Wash off next morning.
- Mix 1 teaspoon lime juice with 1 teaspoon garlic (lahasun) paste and apply on the head.
- Grind 7 to 8 almond (badam) kernels with 1 to 2 teaspoons lime juice and apply on the hair.

Dandruff

- Put about 21 leaves of tulsi and 10 gms. of Aanwala Churna in a big bowl. Add a little of water to make a paste of them. Apply it evenly on your head and allow it to dry. Then wash it with cold water. This will prevent hair loss and clear dandruff also.
- Mix equal quantities of dried curry leaves (curry patta) lime peel (nimbu ka chilka). Shikakai, fenugreek seeds (methi daana and green gram moong saboot) and grind them finely. Store and use as a substitute for soap or shampoo.
- Apply fenugrek (methi) seeds, grind with some water and paste it on the head. Allow to soak at least for 40 minutes before washing. Use every morning for a month.
- Soak 2 tablespoon fenugreek seeds (methi daana) in water overnight. In the morning grind into a fine paste. Apply all over scalp and leave for 1/2 an hour. Wash with Shikakai or mild shampoo.
- Boil a handful of neem leaves in 4 teacups of water. After cooling and filtering use for rinsing hair.

Mental Disorders

Mental ailments do not mean that a person is declare mad or mentally unfit. There are several other problems in day-to -day activities which are related to mental disorders.

FAINTING

Fainting is a sudden brief loss of consciousness caused by a lowering of blood pressure to the brain. Faining may result from physical or emotional causes. Common causative factors are blood loss, dehydration, pain, fright, shock, becoming overheated, exhaustion, arrhythmias of the heart, overexertion, and hyperventilation.

Symptoms

Sudden loss of consciousness with collapse.

Complications

Fainting is usually brief and causes no harm other than the trauma from falling. Fainting may be a symptom of a more serious problem such as shock, head injury, heart attack, stroke or brain tumor. If pulse or breathing are absent, perform CPR (cardio-pulmonary resuscitation) immediately and have someone call for emergency medical assistance. If pulse and respiration are normal, but the person doesn't regain consciousness within a few minutes, seek immediate medical attention.

Homoeopathic Medicines

☞ In cases of fainting due to an extreme fright, give Aconite first.

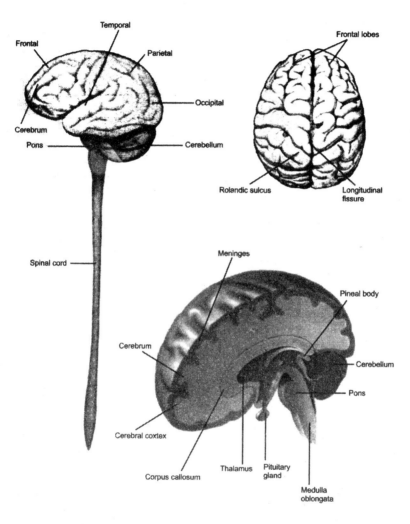

☞ For fainting following an accident or trauma, always give Arnica first.

☞ For fainting from hypothermia or drowning, give Carbo vegetabilis first, then consider Veratrum album.

☞ If the person has fainted follows excitement, give Coffea.

☞ For fainting from stage fright, Gelsemium is the best choice.

☞ Fainting from grief requires Ignatia.

☞ Hysterical fainting calls for Moschus.

Other Self Care Suggestions

☞ Make sure the person has a clear airway.

☞ A cold washcloth on the forehead may help revive the person.

☞ Moisten the lips or tongue with a few drops of Bach Flower Essence Rescue Remedy; it will often work quickly to help revive the person.

☞ Make sure the person has fainted, rather than having suffered a serious injury or heart attack, before moving him.

DIZZINESS

Dizziness is a symptom more than an illness, but it is nonetheless quite annoying and can be debilitating. Dizziness may accompany fever, headache, and nausea in acute illnesses. It is also present with fainting, motion sickness and loss of balance.

Symptoms

Dizziness is often described as a loss of orientation, loss of balance and visual disturbance, often with a "lightheaded" feeling or a sensation of the room spinning. Nausea and vomiting often accompany the dizzy feeling.

Complications

Dizziness may precede loss of consciousness and falling. It may be a symptom of more chronic, serious undelying problems with the endocrine or nervous system or the inner ear, such as hypothyroidism, multiple sclerosis, brain tumors, and meniere's disease. Dizziness may also come from breathing chemical fumes or from alcohol intoxication. Prolonged or recurrent dizziness should be diagnosed by a qualified homoeopath or other qualified healthcare practitioner.

Homoeopathic Medicines

☞ If the dizziness follows a fright or shock, give Aconite.

☞ Give Gelsemium for dizziness due to fright.

☞ When the dizziness is from motion or motion sickness, consider Bryonia or Cocculus first.

☞ Give Bryonia if the patient is very irritable, dry and thirsty and talks of business or wants to go home.

☞ If the dizziness is definitely from riding in a car or airplane or watching moving objects, give Cocculus.

☞ If the dizziness is associated with paralysis or weakness of the legs, you can try Conium first, but also see a homoeopath as soon as possible.

☞ If the dizziness is associated with overall weakness, exhaustion, and dullness of mind, give Gelsemium.

If the dizziness is worse during the menstrual period, when looking upward or from sitting down, in a weepy, clingy person who is worse in a warm, stuffy room, give Pulsatilla.

Self Care and Home Remedies

☞ Hold on to something to prevent falling.

☞ Do not drive or operate machinery while dizzy.

☞ Pick one point and look at it for orientation and balance.

☞ Sit or lie down; close your eyes.

GRIEF

Grief is an emotional reaction to loss and disappointment, such as the loss of a loved one, the breaking up of a relationship, or losing a job.

Symptoms

Grief is characterized by weeping, wailing, sobbing, sighing, withdrawal, and depression. Rational thinking is usually overcome by emotion during acute grief.

Complications

People who are grief stricken may become seriously depressed and even suicidal. If the person makes serious statements about suicide or makes any plans or attempts, emergency psychiatric intervention may be necessary.

Homoeopathic Medicines

☞ Ignatia is the first medicine to think of in acute grief. If there is lots of sobbing and sighing and the person is hysterical give Ignatia.

☞ Natrum muriaticum is useful when the person is withdrawn, hides her tears from others, and desires salty food.

☞ Phosphoric acid should be given when the person is completely exhausted and apathetic after grief or hearing bad news.

Self Care and Home Remedies

☞ Confide your feelings to friends and family or a qualified therapist or spiritual counsellor.

☞ Do not spend too much time alone.

☞ Let yourself cry until it passes on its own.

☞ Try not to dwell too much on the past, guilt, and regrets.

☞ Let the person or situation go, and move on with your life as soon as you are ready.

☞ Do something special for yourself to get your mind off your grief for a time.

☞ Do something to help someone else who needs it.

INSOMNIA

Insomnia is difficulty in falling asleep or staying asleep, to the point that it interferes with getting adequate rest. Insomnia may be caused by emotional distress, worry, nervous tension, too much thinking, pain, drugs, caffeine, overeating, or environments that are not conducive to sleeping.

Symptoms

People with insomnia either can't get to sleep, or they sleep too lightly and awaken too early or too frequently. They often feel tired in the morning upon waking, and do not dream normally.

Lack of sleep contributes to irritability, stress, poor performance at school or work, and a greater tendency to make mistakes or have accidents. People with chrnoic insomnia may become irritable or depressed.

Complications

An occasional lost night of sleep will not cause much difficulty, but chronic insomnia can take its toll on one's health. Sleep deprivation impacts the proper functioning of the immune system and decreases overall alertness and mental functioning.

Homoeopathic Medicines

- ☞ If the person can't sleep following a terrifying experience, the medicine is Aconite.
- ☞ For insomnia that begins right after a financial crisis, give Arsenicum album.
- ☞ For someone who sits up in bed wide awake at 3:00 A.M., think of Coffee.
- ☞ Coffea and chamomilla can be helpful for sleep lessness due to hypersensitivity to pain.
- ☞ For inability to sleep because of anticipation or stage fright, Gelsemium fits best.

☞ If the insomnia began during a period of grieving after the death of a loved one, the best medicine is Ignatia.

☞ People who wake at 3:00 A.M. worrying about business often benefit from Nux vomica.

Self Care and Home Remedies

Drink a cup of warm milk, containing the amino acid tryptophan, one half hour before bedtime.

☞ Equal parts of valerian root, skullcap, passionflower, and hops is a useful herbal sleep formula. Take thirty drops of tincture in warm water one half hour before bedtime or every two hours as needed.

☞ Take an hour of quiet time or relaxation without noise or entertainment before going to bed.

☞ Lie on the right side with arm outstretched to induce sleep more rapidly.

☞ Do alternate nostril breathing for five minutes at bedtime. Close the right nostril with your thumb pressed to the side of your nose. Inhale slowly through the left nostril. With your middle finger close the left nostril, release your thumb to open the right and exhale, Inhale through the right. Then close the right nostril and exhale through the left. Inhale slowly through the left and switch again, exhaling through the right. Continue for three to ten minutes.

HEADACHE

Headache is simply pain in the head. It is more a symptom than a disease. Various kinds of headaches can occur, including tension headaches, migraine headaches and cluster headaches.

Symptoms

The pain of headaches may be localised, or may involve the entire head. It often begins in one place and extends to another.

Many types of pain may occur, such as throbbing, bursting, aching, hammering, and so on. Migraine headaches are often one-sided; they arise from a circulatory problem, and involve visual disturbances, vomiting, and great sensitivity to noise, light, and jarring. Tension headaches often result from increased stress. Headaches in women may have a hormonal component.

Complications

Most headaches resolve on their own over time. Headaches that are very painful, persistent or recurrent may indicate a more serious underlying condition such as a brain tumor or brain aneurysm. Headaches may accompany serious acute illnesses, such as meningitis, strep throat, or other conditions with high fever. If you have very severe or persistent headaches, see a medical professional so that your condition may be properly diagnosed.

Homoeopathic Medicines

☞ Headaches that are worse from the sun: Belladonna, Glonoine, Natrum Muriaticum, Sanguinaria.

☞ Lack of thirst with the headache: Belladonna, Gelsemium.

☞ Right sided headaches: Belladonna, Iris, Sanguinaria.

☞ Migraine headaches: Belladonna, Natrum muriaticum, Iris, Sanguinaria.

☞ Throbbing headaches: Belladonna, Glonoine, Sanguinaria.

☞ Sensitivitiy to light, noise, jarring: Belladonna, Sanguinaria.

☞ Very thirsty with the headache: Belladonna, Bryonia.

☞ Left sided headaches: Bryonia.

☞ Headaches made worse by motion: Bryonia.

☞ Bursting headaches: Bryonia, Glonoine.

☞ Dizzy, drowsy, droopy, and dull: Gelsemium.

☞ Migraine headaches with visual disturbances: Iris.

☞ Headaches from stomach problems: Iris, Sanguinaria.

☞ Headaches with a lot of vomiting: Iris, Sanguinaria.

☞ Migraines with herpes: Natrum muriaticum, Iris.

☞ Burning headaches like a hot wire or poker: Spigelia.

Self Care and Home Remedies

☞ Wrap a cold, wet cloth around your head or use an ice pack while you put your hands and feet in hot water.

☞ Lie down in a dark, quiet place.

☞ Play soft, soothing music.

☞ Do deep, slow breathing.

☞ Take a hot bath with one cup of Epsom salts.

☞ Massage your scalp and the trigger points on your neck and shoulders.

☞ Press deeply on the two points just below the flat bone at the back of the skull about two inches to either side of the centre. Release when the pain goes away.

SHOCK

Shock is inadequate circulation of blood and oxygen to organs or tissues because of blood loss or dehydration, weak action of the heart, or dilation of the peripheral blood vessels.

Septic shock comes from bacterial infection. Anaphylactic shock comes from allergic reactions. Electric shock comes from exposure to live electric current of lightning.

Symptoms

The person is lethargic, sleepy, and confused. Hands and feet are clammy and pale or blue. The pulse and breathing are rapid and weak. In septic shock, fever and chills are usually present. Symptoms of anaphylactic shock include agitation, flushing, heart palpitations, numbness, itching, difficult breathing, hives, swelling, coughing, and sneezing followed by the general symptoms of shock. Electric shock may cause severe muscle contractions, loss of consciousness, heart palpitations or heart failure, and cessation of breathing; burns may also occur.

Complications

Shock is a medical emergency and can lead rapidly to death. Apply first aid measures immediately and call ambulance for emergency medical aid. Keep the person warm, raise his or her legs slightly, stop any blood loss with direct pressure if possible, check the person's airway and breathing, and give CPR (cardio pulmonary resuscitation) if necessary. Do not give anything by mouth that must be swallowed. (Homoeopathic medicines may be dissolved in a small amount of water; a few drops on the tongue are sufficient for a dose.) Turn the head to allow the person to vomit if needed. Hospitalisation is strongly recommended as intravenous fluids, drugs, or surgery may be needed depending on the cause of the shock.

Homoeopathic Medicines

☞ Give Aconite for shock from fright, panic, or emotional causes.

☞ Arnica is very useful for shock from traumatic injuries and blood loss.

☞ Camphora is used for people who are extremely cold and worse from cold, but who paradoxically want cold drinks and to be uncovered.

☞ Carbo vegetabilisis the best medicine for acute shock when the person feels short of breath and wants to be fanned and cooled off.

☞ Carbolic acid is used in anaphylactic shock, especially from a bee sting.

☞ China is very good for shock from loss of bodily fluids, as in dehydration and blood loss.

☞ Veratrum album is good for shock after excessive vomiting, diarrhea, or blood loss.

Self Care and Home Remedies

As shock is a medical emergency, self care and home remedies have been avoided.

■

(13)

Ayurvedic Cure of Nervous Disorders and Vertigo

Vertigo is a disorder related to several nervous disorders. Consider it seriously.

- Steep 1 teaspoon each dried amla powder and coriander seeds (saboot dhania) in water overnight. Strain and drink next morning. To improve the flavour, sugar can be added. Repeat for a few days.
- Heat 2 tablespoon sesame oil (til ka tel). Mix in 1/2 teaspoon each finely powdered cardamom (chhoti illachi) and cinnamon (dalchini). Apply this on head.
- Mix 7 to 8 almonds with 7 to 8 kernels of pumpkin (kaddu) seeds, 1 teaspoon poppy seeds (khuskhus) and 3 tablespoons wheat. Soak in water overnight. Next morning, remove the outer skin of the almonds and grind together into a fine paste. Heat separately 2 teaspoons ghee and fry 1/2 teaspoon cloves (laung). Add the paste to it along with some milk and boil the whole mixture. Sweeten with sugar and drink everyday for a few days.

DEPRESSION

- Boil 1/4 teaspoon powdered cardamom (chhoti illaichi) seeds in thin tea water and drink.
- Mix 1/8 teaspoon nutmeg (jaiphal) powder with 1 tablespoon freshly extracted amla juice. Take 3 times a day.

NERVOUSNESS

- Apply fresh lime juice on the head. Massage well before showering off.
- Steep 1 tablespoon mint (pudina) leaves in 1 cup of water for 30 minutes. Drink the infusion, do not boil.

MEMORY IMPROVEMENT

- Take a mixture of 1 teaspoon honey and a pinch of finely powdered cinnamon (dalchini) every night regularly.
- Take 1/2 teaspoon black cumin (kala jeera) powder and mix it with honey. Eat small quantities of it twice a day.
- Mix 1 teaspoon each amla root powder and white sesame seeds (safed til) powder. Add 1 teaspoon honey and eat everyday for a few days.
- Akhrot (Walnut) and Almonds are good for memory. Take with milk in early morning.

EPILEPSY

- Rub tulsi juice over your body everyday after taking bath.
- Keep the blossoms of tulsi inside the fold of your hanky every time. At the time of attack smell the blossom deeply.
- If the attack makes one unconscious, grind 11 leaves of tulsi, add a little salt to it and put a few drops of this juice in the patient's nostrils. He would immediately regain his consciousness. Keep a tulsi plant in your varanda or somewhere near your bedroom.

HYSTERIA

- If the hysteric effect be due to excess of phlegm in the body, make the patient smell tulsi leaves and drink 5 tulsi leaves juice.

- If it is caused by the excessive heat going to the head, grind five tulsi leaves and five black pepper by mixing them in water and make the patient drink this water every morning and evening for a week's time. Then hysteria will be cured.

MIGRAINE

- Get a small bunch of tulsi blossom, dry in the shade and grind it in powder form. Just take two gms. of it mix about half a spoonful of honey to it and make the person lick it. It is very efficacious treatment. In case you feel like, have another dose for a total cure.

HEADACHE

- Roast some dry ajwain on a tawa. Keep it tightly it in a muslin bag and sniff frequently.
- Make a paste of 2-3 powdered cloves (laung) and salt. Apply this paste on the forehead.
- Tulsi Tea: Mix 8-10 basil (tulsi) leaves, 1/2" piece ginger (adrak), 7 black pepper corns (saboot kali mirchi) powdered coarsely with 1 large cup (200 ml) water. Boil for 2 minutes. Remove from heat, cover and keep for 2-3 minutes. Strain, add boiled milk, sugar and drink warm. Lie down covering yourself with a sheet for 5-10 minutes. It is very helpful in headaches, cold, indigestion. Drink 2-3 times a day. For children reduce quantity to half.
- A ripe apple, after removing the upper rind and the inner hard portion should be taken with a litle salt every morning on an empty stomach. Continue for a week. This yields good results even in case of chronic headaches.
- Mix 1 teaspoon finely grind cinnamon (dalchini) in 1 teaspoon water and apply on the forehead. It is very effective in headache due to exposure to cold air.

- Crush an onion and apply the paste on the head.
- Grind 10-15 tulsi leaves with 4 cloves (laung) and 1 teaspoon dried ginger (sonth) into a paste and apply.

HEADACHE ON THE SIDE

- Powder equal quantities of liquorice (mulathi) and cumin (jeera). Take 1/4 teaspoon everyday along with 1 teaspoon honey for a month.
- Mix 1 teaspoon each of the following powders and store: camphor (kapoor), nutmeg (jaiphal), cardamom (chhoti illaichi) and cloves (laung). Take 2 pinches with warm water.

HEAD HEAVINESS

- Grind the fresh amla fruits into a fine paste and apply on affected parts.
- Grind 2 to 3 cloves (laung) into a fine paste along with 1/2 teaspoon dried ginger (sonth) and apply on nose, forehead etc.

HEMICRANIA (ADHASISI)

- When chronic cold makes the extra phlegm block half of the head, this trouble surfaces. Take a smokeless but hot cowdung cake (Upala) and throw grind turmeric powder over it. It will emit large clouds of smoke. Just inhale this smoke which will make you cough and sneeze and all the blocked phlegm will be expectorated through them. Besides, this, put water turmeric's luke-warm solution in the opposite ear you have this trouble in.

HEADACHE DUE TO EXPOSURE TO COLD AIR

- Mix 1 teaspoon finely grind cinnamon (dalchini) in 1 teaspoon water and apply on the affected parts.

■

Male and Female Disorders

In our society we are not aware about sexual disorders. We hesitate in about such disorders to even the doctors. If there is any problem we should not hesitate in having a proper advice from a genuine person like qualified doctor.

MALE DISORDERS

IMPOTENCY

Why Impotence Shouldn't Be Ignored?

The percentage of men suffering from E.D. (Erectile Dysfunction i.e. Impotency) is very high in our society, but for obvious reasons they don't come forward and continue to suffer, despite having strong sexual desires. Imagine what it must be like not being able to have physical relations for 12 to 15 years !

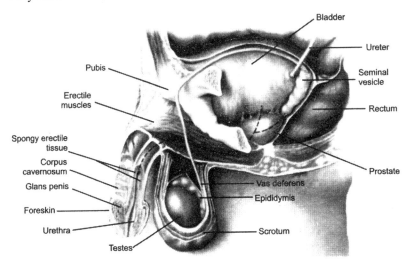

119

Anyway, more and more research and articles and support groups are required to address this problem, which has assumed massive proportions. After all, the fitness of our apparatus is very necessary for keeping the other half of the society happy!

The Culprit in Your Case

After taking a detailed history with special reference etc. medical problems and lifestyle habits, your andrologist/urologist will administer these tests:

- The Nocturnal Penile Turnescense Test in which a computer is attached to the penis at night, to check for erection.
- Intra Penile Injections increase the blood flow to the penis and result in an erection which is observed and rate.
- A Penile Ultra Sound Colour Doppler visualises the blood vessels in the penis.

Mind or Matter?

It is Psychological if
- you wake up with an early morning or middle-of-the-night erection
- you have had satisfactory interactive intercourse
- you masturbate perfectly well
- your problem occurred suddenly

It is Physical if
- your erection is feeble and does not strengthen even while you sleep, wake up in the morning, or masturbate
- you fail again and again
- the onset is gradual

Irksome Illnesses

By far the most common illnesses that cause impotence is diabetes; over half of all older diabetics have or will have erectile difficulties; 20 percent of hypertensive can suffer, too.

Other culprits are high cholesterol, spinal injury, pelvic surgery, excessive drinking and smoking which damage the blood vessels.

Incidentally the latest research shows that if you suffer from vascular erectile dysfunction, It is wise to have a cardiac check up, because a link has been established between furred arteries of the penis and faculty arteries of the heart.

With added medical awareness, prescribed drugs such as antihistamines and antidepressants are being held responsible for only 10 percent of the cases. Harmon imbalances are even rarer, account for a more 1 percent.

Something For Everyone

Treatments for impotence are available for every age, condition, need, preference or social situation.

FAMOUS HOMOEOPATHIC MEDICINES

Lycopodium

It is the most famous homoeopathic medicine. Famous serologist of U.S.A. Dr. Nash M.D. Says that if taken in proper dose this drug not only makes youth robust filled with abundant semen, it even revitalise the sexual potency of the old persons. The effect of the medicine is not temporary but permanent one, hence it should be administered in fixed intervals of time. This medicine is available in various potencies, from 200 to 10000 or even of one lakh potency. The higher the potency the better would be the results. But it is advisable that these medicines should be taken after proper medical advice. Or else they create quite serious complications. This medicine is especially recommended for those strayed youth who ruin their sexual potency by constant use of their male organ. In fact, this medicine should be taken by increasing its potency gradually. The medicine of 200 potency should be given on empty stomach to the patient and the next dose of higher potency, after one full week. The same way the potency should be increased from 1000 to the dose of the desired potency when the affliction is cured.

Phosphoric Acid

It is also a wonder homoeopathic drug to cure sexual weakness. The constant malpractice result in the patient's face becoming pale and sallow, eyes sunken in the sockets and constant complaints of pain in the waist. The afflicted person's semen also becomes very thin and often passes out with urine while passing stool. This medicine is also good for those patients afflicted with diabetes. It not only enhances the physical power of the patient but makes him very strong mentally also. This medicine is to be administered mixed with three to five drops of mother tincture diluted with 25 to 30 gms. of water. Ask the patient to have the medicine before taking his meal. Phosphoric acid is a powerful drug and should not be administered on empty stomach.

Avenasativa

The cautious use of this celebrated medicine administered mixed with five to six drops of mother tincture is an unfailing remedy for all the sexual weakness. A timid listless boy turns into a robust man by the use of this medicine. It not only strengthens the user's body but increases the efficiency of his mental faculties.

Caution

All these medicines are to be taken after proper medical advice. Don't rush to take them without consulting some good homoeopathic physician. Other good remedies are caladium, conium, staphysagria, and selenium.

FEMALE DISORDERS

Dysmenorrhoea (Menstrual Cramps)

This is painful menstruation colicky pain during menses.

Homoeopathic Medicines

- ☞ If there is heavy, bright red bleeding, gushing and throbbing pain, look first at Belladonna.
- ☞ If the pain is lessened by heat and pressure, think first of Magnesia phosphorica, then of Colocynthis.
- ☞ For pain is very intense and the woman is terribly angry and inconsolable, look at Chamomilla.
- ☞ If the woman feels better when drawing her knees up to her chest, give Colocynthis.
- ☞ If the pain began after anger, think of Nux vomica, Colocynthis, and Belladonna.
- ☞ If the pain came on after too much alcohol or rich food, give Nux vomica.

Self Care and Home Remedies

- ☞ Alternating hot and cold sitz baths: soak in tub of moderately hot water for five minutes, then in a tub of cold water up to the navel with knees bent for one minute. Alternate two to three times.

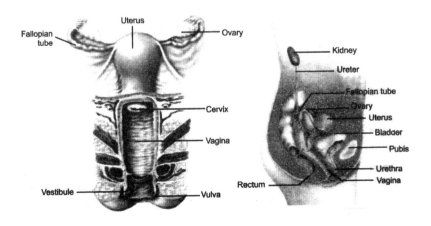

☞ Walking stretching and other physical exercise can sometimes help.

☞ For muscle cramps, Calcium and Magnesium can help.

☞ Take Viburnum tincture: one half teaspoon every hour, up to six doses. The dosage for capsules depends on the specific product.

☞ A heating pad is often helpful.

☞ Castor oil packs to the abdomen with a heating pad can sometimes relieve discomfort.

☞ Avoid caffeine and salt premenstrually.

PAIN REDUCES PLEASURE

After my children were born, I have not enjoyed sex at all. I am protected against getting pregnant again so I feel that's not a problem. Also, I enjoyed sex a lot before children. Sometimes I think its all in my head, that if I could let myself enjoy it I wouldn't feel any pain; yet I know there's something wrong down then. My gynaecologist has not been able to figure anything out.

This kind of report typifies a woman who is eager for a sexual experience but is finding each encounter to be more and more negative because of the intense pain she experiences during each sexual act. Pain during intercourse is technically called dyspareunia. It has a number of different sources. Whatever the source, when pain is experienced sexual enjoyment will be greatly reduced if not eliminated altogether.

PAIN AND THE NEW BRIDE

For the new bride who is a virgin it is not surprising if there is a small amount of pain. Most women experience at least a little. This can be due to the opening in the hymen being tight and small. In the great majority of situations it is due to a ˜bination of newne, excitement and anxiety which prevents woman from relaxing. When the necessary physical changes do not take place (the opening up and laying flat of the majora lips, plus lubrication), then entry is going to be more difficult and pain more intense. Entry under these conditions increases the pain and reduces the possibility of pleasure. Once the woman feels pain, tension is likely to set in. This tension will inhibit arousal and block any kind of release. While many couples begin in this way they usually get past the sequence quite quickly. But the sequence can be avoided to begin with.

If you are an engaged couple or if you counsel engaged couples, attending to a few small details will reduce much of the anxiety and potential for pain. First six weeks to two months before the wedding date the woman should be examined by gynaecologist or qualified general practitioner. In this experience the doctor should be able to communicate to her whether her physical anatomy is normal and whether there are any particular barriers of which she should be aware. The couple and the physician should discuss birth control methods.

In the weeks before the marriage, every time the bride-to-be takes a bath she should use her fingers to stretch the hymen until she can insert three fingers into the vagina and pull it apart slightly. This stretching procedure will prepare the vagina for entry and will also help the woman become familiar with some of the sensations of having the vagina stretched. As the wedding comes closer this might be done several times a day.

The couple should be encouraged to take along a lubricant that is not sticky (not Vaseline). K-Y jelly or Lubrifax are recommended for genital use. For use over the whole body as well as genitally, a nonallergic lotion without lanolin such as Allercreme is good. The couple should plan to use the lubricant for all entry experiences, whether they think they need it or not. The lubricant protects the woman. In case she dries up during the excitement. It also provides a distraction from the focus on the entry. A small amount of lubricant should be applied to the head and ridge of the penis and to the opening of the vagina.

A final word of instruction to the new bride and groom is to move slowly. No matter how many times they tell themselves to proceed slowly they will still most likely move ahead too quickly. If a couple can plan to move into their first experience with a great deal of gentleness, patience, ease, and relaxation, they are most likely to create a positive beginning to a life of loving.

STRESS BRINGS PAIN

All of us show our tension in our own unique way. Some women, as they experience tension surrounding the sexual experience, will tend to tighten up their genital muscles involuntarily. In fact, they may not even be aware that the tensing is happening. Since this is counterproductive to a fulfilling and releasing sexual experience, It is not surprising that these women end up frustrated. But even more than the frustration as a result of the tension, they may experience palm. For example, if the tightening occurs before entry it may cause pain upon entry. Sharp, spasmodic contractions after entry may also cause pain. The extreme form of this tension is called vaginismus.

Vaginimus is the involuntary tightening of the muscles. In the outer third of the vagina which prevents the insertion of the penis. This contraction can be so severe that it is impossible to insert even your small finger. It can become a permanent state rather than just occurring as a result of the initiation of sex play. Because it is impossible for the man to enter, vaginismus is easily identified. Should this be your situation, consult a gynaecologist immediately and specifically explain your situation. If he or she is not familiar with the usual treatment procedures ask for a referral either to another physician or to a sex therapist. This professional must be competent to guide you in the use of a series of dilators which are graduated in size and designed to eliminate these involuntary spasms. Be encouraged that this condition is extremely responsive to treatment in a relatively brief period of time. However, there should be some attempt also to understand the events leading to the vaginismus so that his pattern will not be repeated.

Another source of pain due to tension occurs with lack of release. When a woman does not experience an orgasm, she may sense some painful sensations in the lower abdominal area and the lower back. As she has become aroused the whole reproductive system, including the vaginal area and the uterus has become congested with blood in preparation for the organic release. The contractions of the orgasm are designed to release it's congestion, so that the blood which has fined the cavities can be drained. When there is an orgasm this process provides a great deal of pleasure. When the woman does not experience release, the whole pelvic area remains engorged, which may cause chronic pain. This pain is usually not intense, but is a dull, throbbing ache similar to lower back pain. The difference is that it feels like it is further inside the body. Obviously the best remedy for this pain is for a woman to allow herself to experience orgasm. In consulting a physician or therapist it is crucial to identify when the pain occurs and thus determine if it is the result of lack of orgasmic release.

PHYSICALLY BASED PAIN

Infections and irritations will obviously reduce pleasure. Whether the infection is in the external genitalia, causing pain during clitoral stimulation, or is inside the vagina, causing pain during intercourse, it will hinder freedom and enjoyment. Any kind of infection should immediately be dealt with by a physician. Sexual activity should be limited according to the instruction of the physician. Sometimes an infection provides the opportunity for the couple to focus on the rest of the body for those often bypassed, special pleasures. Just because there is an infection does not mean the couple should abstain from all sexual activity. If it is comfortable for both, the man can be stimulated to orgasm at the end of a total body experience without ever having contact with the woman's genitals.

Irritations are troublesome because there is no specific identifiable disease present. Yet an irritated vaginal opening or vaginal barrel can cause as much distress and pain during love-making as an infection. The best antidote to irritation is the generous use of a lubricant. Some women experience a thinning of the vaginal walls. Sometimes this happens with age, particularly around the time of menopause because of a reduction of estrogen. If the walls of your vagina are thinning, again consult a physician to determine the cause and then always use a lubricant to reduce friction. Even if the walls of the vagina are becoming thin, pleasurable activity need not cease.

Pain can also be the result of tears either in the opening of the vagina or small cuts (fissures) inside the vagina itself. Tears in the hymen usually cause pain on entry. Some women can identify pain at a very specific spot inside the vagina. Their report usually goes something like this: "It feels as if it is in the lower left-hand corner about an inch inside the vagina and it hurts exactly the same way every time. I feel I can even reach in and put my finger on it". When the pain is this specific, it is usually not the result of tension or the thinning of the vaginal walls but rather the result of a small tear inside the vagina. Because of continued sexual activity and the moist environ-ment, healing is slow. When consulting a physician be sure to identify the exact location of the pain. Show the doctor so that he can carefully warn it and determine the nature of the problem. As a rule these tears can be treated with an ointment.

Some women report pain only during deep thrusting. There are three main sources of this kind of pain. The most commonly reported discomfort is the result of a lipped or retroverted uterus. When the muscles that suspend the uterus are weakened, the uterus drops so that the cervix, the opening to the uterus falls into the upper end of the vagina. As deep thrusting occurs the penis strikes the cervix, causing sharp, stabbing pain. It may cause a woman to cry out. Relief can be found immediately by a slight shift in position. For many women a small pillow or folded towel under the lower back (if she is under the man) will shift the uterus enough so that deep thrusting can be enjoyed.

Other internal pathologies such as endometriosis or a misplaced IUD can also cause pain upon deep thrusting.

Finally, there may be pain as an outgrowth of trauma from childbirth. One such pain occurs in the sensitive scars from the episiotomy, the incision that is made between the vagina and the rectum to assist the birth process. There also may be tears in the ligaments that hold the uterus in place, in the vaginal wall or around the opening of the vagina. Tears are more likely to occur with a difficult birth. This was true for us after the breech (feet first) delivery of our first child. For those resuming sexual activity after the birth of a child we would issue the same encouragement given to the newly married couple: move carefully and slowly, haste will only hurt; be generous with the lubricant.

MANAGING PAIN

Whenever you experience pain, the first thing you should do is talk about it with your husband. Never grit your teeth and bear it. Define exactly where the pain is located and when in the love-making process it occurs. Even before you get to the physician you may be able to avoid the situations that cause the pain if you guide the penis for entry and shift positions to make adjustments. Except for pain from deep thrusting, lubrication will almost always reduce some of the intensity, even if it is from an infection. Then, discover what is pleasurable and focus on that for the time being. Avoiding entry for a few love-making sessions may be necessary. It is important not to continue the activity that triggers the pain. Whenever a negative sensation like pain is associated with a pleasurable activity like sexual play or intercourse, the pleasurable event will begin to take on the negative feelings. Even after the physical reason for the pain has healed, a woman may continue to tense up or avoid the sexual activity that was linked with the pain. Her pulling away and tightening up has become a conditioned response. Sometimes the pain will continue because of the tension. In dealing with this, use the same approach as you would for any emotional hesitancy or avoidance. Begin gradually, letting the woman take the lead until the tension concerning the pain has been reduced.

An increasing number of women, particularly young women, are reporting pain during intercourse. If you are among these, seek help after talking about it with your partner. Pain does not have to be tolerated. In fact, pain cannot be allowed to continue if you are going to enjoy sexual pleasure.

MORNING SICKNESS

Morning sickness occurs most commonly in the first three months of pregnancy, but may persist in some cases until the baby is born. It is commonly experienced in the morning, but may last throughout the day or come at different times.

Symptoms

Terrible nausea with aversion to the sight and smell of food are usual symptoms. Vomiting may be pronounced, with inability to kep most food and beverages down.

Complications

Apart from the discomfort and inconvenience, the main complication of prolonged morning sickness is malnutrition and failure of the mother to gain appropriate weight, with subsequent low birth weight and congenital health problems for the child. Hyperemesis gravidarum- severe uncontrollable vomiting in pregnancy, often associated with liver disease- may cause dehydration and acidosis, requiring hospitalisation and intravenous fluids.

Homoeopathic Medicines

☞ The most common medicines for morning sickness are Sepia and Colchicum.

☞ When aversion to the smell of food is strongest, consider Colchicum first.

☞ For the worst vomiting, use Ipecac, and for the most deathly nausea, use Tabacum.

☞ When aversion to sex is a strong symptom, consider Sepia or Kreosotum.

☞ Sepia is for conditions that are made much better by vigorous exercise or dancing, which separates it from the motion sickness medicines such as Tabacum and Cocculus; the latter two are appropriate for conditions that are made much worse by motion.

☞ Veratrum is the medicine if the woman is very cold, has vomiting and diarrhea and desires fruit, ice, and sour foods such as pickles or lemons.

Self Care and Home Remedies

☞ Eat small amounts of food frequently.

☞ Eat before getting up in the morning.

☞ Eat Saltine crackers to help relieve the nausea.

☞ Eat bland foods such as broth, rice, and pasta.

☞ Tea and toast are usually well tolerated.

☞ Sipping ginger root tea can help relieve nausea. Use a one quarterinch slice of ginger root boiled in a cup of water for fifteen minutes.

☞ Many herbs, such as pennyroyal, need to be avoided during pregnancy.

☞ Stimulating Stomach, an acupressure point in the soft place below the knee and to the outside of the leg where the tibia and fibula bones meet, often relieves nausea. Use firm rotary pressure on the spot for a few seconds. Repeat when needed.

THRUSH

Thrush is a yeast infection of the mucous membranes inside the mouth. It is common in infants, people who have been treated with antibiotics, and people with compromised immune systems, as in AIDS.

Symptoms

There are creamy white patches on the tongue or the mucous membranes of the mouth that can be scraped off.

Complications

None, unless the thrush continues for a long time and turns into a systemic yeast infection.

Homoeopathic Medicines

☞ By far the most common medicine for thrush is Borax, especially if there are also canker sores.

☞ If there is bad smelling breath, perspiration, and body odor, give Mercurius.

☞ If the tongue burns and has a thick furry coating, consider Sulphur.

Self Care and Home Remedies

☞ If the nursing baby had thrush, the mother should also be treated if she has a breast infection.

☞ Acidophilus or unsweetened yogurt can help reestablish healthy intestinal flora.

☞ Avoid eating anything sweet, since yeast thrives on sugar.

☞ The most common treatment for thrush in many parts of the world is topical gentian violet, but it stains and is generally unnecessary due to the effectivenenss of homoeopathy.

VAGINITIS

Vaginitis is an inflammation of the mucous membranes of the vagina. It may be caused by a viral, bacterial, trichomonal, or yeast infection, or by sexual intercourse, douching, or other irritants such as spermicides, chemicals, or a foreign body in the vagina. Atrophic vaginitis occurs in women past menopause, resulting from a decrease in estrogen levels.

Symptoms

Vaginal discharge is often the main complaint. It may be thick or thin, odorless or offensive. There may also be redness of the vaginal lips and itching, swelling or pain of the vulva, labia and vagina. The intensity varies greatly.

Complications

A culture of the vaginal discharge should be taken to find out the cause of the infection. If gonorrhea, chlamydia, or syphilis are found to be the cause, the diagnosis must be reported to the local public health department and immediate medical attention is required. These three infections are often asymptomatic in women and, if untreated, may lead to infertility.

Homoeopathic Medicines

- ☞ For vaginitis with terrible itching during pregnancy, give Caladium.
- ☞ For vaginal discharges that are terribly abrasing and acrid, give Kreosotum.
- ☞ For vaginitis with a yellowish green creamy discharge in a gentle woman who cries as she tells you about it, Pulsatilla will probably work.
- ☞ If the discharge smells strongly like fish brine, look at Sanicula.
- ☞ If the symptoms occur during menopause and are accompanied by a lack of sex drive, constipation, and irritability, Sepia will be helpful.

Self Care and Home Remedies

☞ The easiest and most effective suggestion: insert one capsule of boric acid into the vagina in the morning, and one capsule of acidophilus at bedtime, for five days. Stop during the menstrual period.

☞ Douche with one tablespoon of white vinegar in a pint of warm water daily for five days. Insert one tablespoon of unsweetened, live culture yogurt after each douche.

☞ If the vaginitis is just on the labia and vulva and is caused by yeast, apply a preparation of half vinegar and half water topically.

☞ Some women insert a clove of garlic, wrapped in cheesecloth or gauze, vaginally for yeast infections.

☞ If there is rawness externally not due to yeast, Calendula cream topically can be helpful.

☞ Insert Vitamin E suppositories into the vagina for vaginal dryness.

☞ Occasionally, one tablespoon of baking soda in a quart of water works better as a douche than acidifying treatments such as vinegar or boric acid.

■

15

Ayurvedic Cure of
Disorders of Male

PHYSICAL WEAKNESS

- Soak 2 or 3 dried figs (anjeer) overnight in 1 cup of water. Eat them along with 1 tablespoon honey the next morning. Continue for a month.
- Fry in 1 tablespoon butter, 2 teaspoons each wheat flour, almond paste and poppy seeds (khuskhus) paste. Eat this along with 1 cup boiled leaves of fenugreek (methi).

Testes Problem

- It there be swelling on the testes or any other problem concerning with testes, apply the paste prepared in the following manner over the testes. Take about 5 gms. each of a camel's dung. Amarbel (easily available in Mango groves), the leaves of Arhar and tulsi leaves, Grind them to a homogeneous paste in a little of cow's urine, when the paste is ready, apply it over the testes thickly. Allow it to dry and remove it in the morning. A week's treatment will cure all troubles connected with the testes.

Venereal Disease (Gonorrhoea)

- Juice of tulsi leaves is very effective to cure all sort of these troubles. Take 5 gms. each of tulsi seeds or dried tulsi leaves, Kalami shora and the grains of small cardamom. Grind them together to powder form. Have this combination (just 1/2 gm.) with 100 gms. Kacchi Lassi (raw milk and water combination). Add water twice the amount of milk. Drink this lassi with that powder thrice or four times a day. But don't add either salt or sugar in the lassi. About a fortnight long this treatment shall get you cured from any sort of veneral disease.

Nocturnal Ejaculation

- Grind the dry ginger and add sugar to it. Have this powder everyday in the morning. First eat the powder (about 10 gms.) daily and wash it down with 100 gms. of milk.
- Take about 5 gms. of misri with 100 gms. of milk in the night or morning.
- Take a glass of cold water as the first thing in the morning after you have cleared your bowels.
- Take mochras, kamarkas, khus-khus (kinds of poppy seeds) and 6 gms. of Bishop's seeds. Grind and sieve them to a powdered form. Take this powder daily with 250 gms. of milk for quick relief.
- A glass of cold water on an empty stomach in the morning is highly recommended. Ten grams of dry corriander grind in water and sweetened with sugar should be taken in the morning.
- Six grams of leafshoots of acacia grind in water also help this condition.
- A sufferer from nocturnal pollutions must take exercise in the evening (before dinner) so that he becomes too tired to dream and has a sound sleep.

Deteriorating Sexual Potency

- Take 30 gms. washed Urad Dal and fry it in pure ghee. Then mix it in 300 gms. of milk and thicken it to kheer form. Then add sugar as required and eat it hot. This kheer is very efficacious to enhance your sexual potency.

- Take white Mossali 25 gms. Isabgol Bhusi 40 gms. and grind and sieve both to get a soft powder. Cook the whole lot in about 300 gms. of milk. Add sugar and have it daily in the night after your dinner to enhance your sexual potency.

- Take 2 teaspoons of amla juice and mix it with two teaspoonfuls each honey and lime juice. Add 1 teacup water and drink on an empty stomach every morning. (Attention: The treatment should continue for at least 120 days to achieve expected results.)

- Boil 1 teaspoon grind fenugreek seeds (methi dana) in a cup of water and drink.

- 1/2 teaspoon ginger (adrak) juice mixed with honey and a semi boiled egg, taken at night.

- Mix 1/4 teaspoon nutmeg (jaiphal) powder in a teaspoon honey and take milk an hour before going to bed.

- Onion seeds (kalaunji) dried and powdered, 1 teaspoon eaten 3 times daily along with sugar or honey.

- Take about 100 gms. of the seeds of radish. Dry them fully then pound them to powder form. Now strain them through a fine but coarse cloth. Start taking 5 gms. of this powder with 100 gms. of butter. If butter is not available, you can have it with cream as well, in about 10 days' time you shall be again virile. But continue the treatment for atleast one month.

- Fry equal quantities of carom (ajwain) seeds and kern of tamarind seeds (imli ke beej) in ghee. Powder th mixture and store in a dry, cool place. Mix 1 teaspo of this powder in a glass of milk along with tablespoon honey. Drink daily at bedtime.

- Soak 8 to 10 almonds and 1 teaspoon rice overnig Remove the outer skin. Grind into a fine paste. Mi: some milk and a pinch of turmeric (haldi) powder. I and drink along with sugar candy (mishri) or ordin sugar to taste.

- Mix ¼ teaspoon saffron (kesar) with milk. Take twice daily.

Premature Ejaculation

- Take 10 gms. pure ghee, 5 gms. honey, grind liquorice 10 gms. Make a paste of all the three and lick it regularly. Wash it down with 250 gms. of milk. Have it after the intercourse.
- Grind dry coriander seeds. mix it with 'missri' and have about 5 gms. of this powder washed down with cold water.
- Take basil seeds 50 gms; sugar 50 gms. and grind and sieve the whole lot. Take just 6 gms. of this powder, and drink it with 100 gms. of milk early in the morning.
- Take the seeds of Lajwanti plant and mix it with equal amount of sugar. Take 5 gms. of this mixture and wash it down with 100 gms. of milk. This combination thickens the semen and stops early ejaculation.

IMPOTENCE

Impotence is a disorder peculiar to males: in females the corresponding disorder is known as frigidity (the absence of sexual desire and a failure to respond to sexual stimulii). Impotence may be defined as the inability to perform the sex act or incomplete performance (premature ejaculation) which leaves the female partner dissatisfied. Impotence may be organic or functional. Among the organic causes are lesions of the external genitals, i.e. a tight foreskin, disturbance of the endocrine glands, such as diminished activity of the gonads (as happens in old age.) diseases of the nervous system, diabetes, alcoholism. Among the psychological factors are ignorance, fear, weakness of sexual desire or a guilt complex which may inhibit the action of the gonads.

It has been found that in a majority of the males suffering from impotence, the reasons are psychological. They may be suffering from a guilt complex because they may have indulged in masturbation, unnatural sex or incest (sexual relations with near kindered) during their early life. Or, they might be always thinking of sex, being in an agitated state of mind all the time and suffer from premature ejaculation. If the reasons for impotence are psychological only a proper psychoanalysis of the patient will help. It could be explained to the sufferer that having masturbated in early life does not sexually incapacitate a male. But after all the psychological methods have been tried, the following remedies should be used:

- In case of spermatorrhoes (ejaculation even without the penis having attained tumescence), tender, seedless pods of Acacia should be dried in the shade and powdered before being mixed with an equal weight of raw sugar. Six grams of it should be taken with milk in the morning.
- Leaf shoots of Banyan tree may be substituted for acacia pods.
- Cotton tree dried in the shade and powdered before mixing it with an equal amount of raw sugar should be taken in 10 grams dose with milk.
- Fifty grams each of Kernels of seeds of Bastard Teak (Dhak) and siris tree finely grind and mixed with 50 gms. of raw sugar should be taken in six grams dose every morning for three weeks to relieve the condition. Fifty grams each of dry amla and mango, ginger, amba, haldi should be powdered and mixed with an equal weight of raw sugar. The daily morning dose is six grams, taken with milk.

■

(16)

Ayurvedic Cure
of Disorders of Females

The female's body is a complexed creation, where there are chances of many disorders. But problems like abortion are self created.

OVARY PROBLEM

Those ladies who have this problem must eat vegetable of beetroot during their meals. If this problem is caused by some vitamin and mineral deficiency, such a diet will cure the problem very soon. All the physicians are unanimous in their choice in prescribing beetroot for such ladies.

Reproductive Weakness

- Boil 1 cup of milk with 1/2 teaspoon pepper powder and to 8 crushed almonds. Take at bedtime.

Lack of Milk in Mother's Breast

- If the mother takes regular beetroot diet even before delivery she is not likely to have this problem. However if she has not done so, she must start drinking beetroot juice as the first thing in the morning and must eat a lot of fresh beetroot as salad. In less than a week this problem will end.

Sexual Underdevelopment in Women

- 6 to 8 almonds, crushed and mixed in 1 cup of milk along with 1 egg yolk, 1/2 teaspoon grind sesame seeds (til) and 1 teaspoon honey. Take once or twice a day.

Sexual Weakness

- Onion seeds (kalaunji) powdered, 1 teaspoon eaten 3 times daily along with sugar or honey.

Easy Delivery of Baby

- Mix 3 teaspoon lime juice, 1/4 teaspoon powdered black pepper and 1 teaspoon honey in 1 cup of water. Drink for 3 months.

Family Planning

Device: The treatment mentioned below is especially meant for the ladies. If the lady during her menses, takes five gms. of grind turmeric and wash it down with water. She would not conceive at all. This treatment is very effective for family planning, when the couple decides not to have an issue, the wife must resort to this treatment. Or you can have copper 's or contraceptive pills. These are the safest methods without any adverse side effects.

Menstrual Disturbance

In cases of scanty discharge of menstrual blood, the main cause should be diagnosed and removed. If it is due to anaemia, the treatment of anaemia is a prerequisite to the treatment of this problem. If it is because of anaemia the treatment given above for anaemia should be adopted to.

- To cure this trouble mix beetroot in water and then squeeze the pieces to convert the whole solution to a homogeneous form. Strain it through a strainer and drink it thrice or four times a day for speedy cure.

Menstrual Pains

- Boil 1 teaspoon saffron in 1/2 cup of water. Let it reduce to become 1 tablespoon. Divide this decoction into three portions and take with equal quantities of water, thrice daily for a couple of days.

Menstruation Delay

- Take 1/2 teaspoon finely grind cinnamon (dalchini) every night along with 1 cup milk.
- Powder 1 teaspoon dried mint (pudina) leaves and take with 1 teaspoon honey, thrice daily.
- 6 to 8 almonds, crushed and mixed in 1 cup milk with 1 egg yolk, 1/2 teaspoon sesame (til) powder and 1teaspoon honey. Take once or twice a day.

Excessive Bleeding in Menstruation

- Grind the fuller's earth and mix it in 250 gms. of water. Soak it overnight. Then drink the sedimented water every morning.
- Take the rind of the Ashok Tree, about 10 gms; boil it in one kg. of milk and 250 gms. of water till the quantitiy is halved. Then cool it and add some mishr to it to sweeten it. Have it in the morning and evening. In about a week's time the disorder shall be set right.
- Grind some bel leaves into a fine paste. Take 1 teaspoon with warm water and drink some cold water as well.
- Grind 10 fresh buds of figs (anjeer) and apply on the lower abdomen below the navel for a few hours. Repeat this frequently.
- Boil 1 tablespoon coriander (dhania) seeds in 2 cups of water till it is reduced to 1 cup. Add sugar to taste and drink when lukewarm. Repeat twice or thrice a day.

Stoppage of Menstruation

- Take about 10 gms. of carrot seed and 20 gms. of jaggery and boil in 500 gms of water till the water i reduced to one third of its normal quantity. Then strain the water and ask the afflicted lady to drink it twice daily, about 2 spoonfuls. In a couple of days the bleeding would commence in the normal cycle.

Take 10 gms. of black til, gokhru 10 gms. and mix both in about 250 gms. of water. Drink the water twice daily, about 2 teaspoonfuls every time.

Morning Sickness

- Mix juice of 15-20 tender curry leaves (curry patta) with 2 teaspoon lime juice and 1 teaspoon sugar. Take in the morning.
- Mix 1/8 teaspoon nutmeg (jaiphal) powder with 1 tablespoon freshly extracted amla juice. Take 3 times a day.
- 1/2 teaspoon ginger (adrak) juice with 1 teaspoon each fresh mint (pudina) juice mixed with a tablespoon of honey, taken frequently.
- Mix 1 teaspoon each fresh juice of mint (pudina) and lime along with 1 tablespoon honey. Take 3 times a day.

Lactation in Mothers

- Mix together 1 teaspoon each cumin (jeera) powder and sugar and take with warm milk after dinner every day for a few days.
- Boil 2 teaspoon cumin (jeera) seed in 1/2 cup water. Filter it. Mix in 1/2 cup milk and 1 teaspoon honey. Drink once a day for a few days.
- Boil 2 teaspoon fennel seeds (saunf) in barley water and take twice or thrice a day.
- Frequently, cook unripe papayas (kacha papita) and eat.
- 1/2 teaspoon finely grind cinnamon (dalchini) taken at night along with 1 cup of milk.

Amenorrhoea

- A week before the period of a women are due, a decoction of six grams of flex seeds, about 250 ml. of water reduced to half through boiling mixed with 20 grams of jaggery and 20 grams of ghee should be taken daily. Alternatively a decoction of ten grams of seeds of carrot and jaggery should be taken for about a week. Another remedy is to boil six grams of baberang (Embelia Ribes) three grams of dry ginger and 20 grams of jaggery in 500 ml. of water till half of it is left. The decoction should be taken for some days. It shows its effect.

- Decoction of 20 grams each of flowers and leaves of the cotton plant (500 ml. of water boiled to half its quantity) mixed with 20 grams of jaggery is also effective in inducing the menstrual flow. Another remedy is to steep 10 grams of black sesame seeds and an equal quantity of small galtrops (Gokhru) in 250 ml. of water and to grind them in the same water. It should be sweetened with sugar and drunk.

Dysmenorrhoea

- One hundred grams of juice of green leaves of black Nightshade (mako) and leaves of Chicory (kasni) should be placed on fire and when it coagulates, it should be strained and drunk after mixing 20 grams of Jaggery with it. Twenty grams of the leaves of the following eight herbs are boiled in water (i) Sambhalu (Indian wild pepper), (ii) Sahingana (horse radish), (iii) Bakayan (Indian Lilac) (iv) Kasni (wild Chicory) (v) Mako (Black Nightshade) (vi) Khatmi (Marsh Mallow), (vii) Narma Kapas (cotton plant) and (viii) Soya (dill). When the leaves are cooked and the water evaporated, they should be fried in sesame oil like any vegetable and tied to the lower abdomen like a poultice. It will deal effectively with inflammation.

- A very helpful remedy for the pain of dysmenorrhoea is a decoction of root of Cotton Tree (18 grams), Telia Geru (6 grams) leaves of Rose Bush (6 grams), Root of Chaulai (6 grams), Gur (24 grams) boiled in 750 ml. of water till one eighth is left. The decocton should be taken for three days continuously. Alternatively, 120 milligrams of the drug may be kept in the vagina to find relief.

Menorrhagia and Metrorrhagia

If there is excessive discharge of blood from the womb during the monthly periods, it is called menorrhagia, but if there is irregularity of menstruation, the condition is called metrorrhagia. The treatment for both the conditions is the same.

- The disorders may be due to the imbalance of the hormones, abnormal growths (Whether benign or malignant) in the uterus may be at the root of excessive or irregular bleeding. In severe cases, bleeding may continue for a long time giving rise to symptoms of prostration like giddiness, constant headaches, pain in the calves and restlessness. Neglect of the condition or ineffective attempts at dealing with it may lead to anaemia of the most severe type. Saraca Indica and Lodhra (symplocos racemasa) are two remedies which have been successfully used by the practitioners of Ayurveda to deal with these conditions. A home remedy is to grind seven leaves of the pomegranate tree and seven grains of rice into a paste and given to the patient for a month twice daily. It acts as a curative as well as a preventive agent.

- Twenty grams of bark of Ashoka tree should be crushed and boiled in 250 ml. of milk and equal amount of water. When half of the liquid is left, it should be strained, sweetened with sugar and drunk. A few days use will put the patient on the road to recovery. Or , equal weight of Pathani Lodh Red Ochre (geru) and Oak Galls (mazu) should be finely powdered and four grams of it taken in the morning and evening with milk.

- Half ripe fruits of the country fig tree (Gular) should be dried in the shade, powdered and mixed with an equal quantity of sugar. Six grams of the powder taken with milk in the morning and evening gives relief. Alternatively, three grams of Rasaut and an equal quantity of shellac should be finely grind together and made into two doses, one to be taken with milk in the morning and evening.

Another wonderful remedy for this condition is Amla. Dry Amla should be soaked in juice of green Amla for three days and then grind into powder. Six grams of this powder taken with cow's milk for some days cures the conditions.

Other remedies recommended are 10 grams each of selkhari (chalk) and geru (red ochre) grind together should be taken in three grams doses thrice daily.

Multani Mitti steeped in water and the supernatant water drunk in the morning is also good for excessive bleeding from the womb. Five grams of bark of kurchi and raw sugar mixed together taken in the morning and evening is also an effective remedy.

Abortion

Take about three to four medium sized radishes and boil them in water. Add 100 gms. water for each radish and boil it by steam. When water becomes dry, squeeze the radish and add soft leaves of radish to it also. Do not add salt. Instead add a little of sugarcandy. The lady should have it twice a day.

Leucorrhoea

It is generally called a 'white discharge' or simply 'the whites'. In reality, leucorrhoea is a state where there is catarrhal discharge from the Vagina's mucous membrane. This is the most agonising disorder for the females and distort their health. It may last a life-time or prolong for sometime and then abate or may appear as and when her health is in poor state.

Leucorrheal Flow

- The discharge is often white, like white portion of an, egg or milk-colour, or else it may be off white, yellow, reddish or pinkish, green or light blue, but in most of the cases, it is odourless and white.
- Flow may stiffen the linen or simply leave back a trace of white powder or scales.
- It may excoriate vulva and thighs and the itching caused is sometime too intense and so much that blood oozes out from the site itched.
- Consistency of discharge varies-from water to consistency of cream, milk, viscous fluid or even albuminous.
- In most cases discharge emanates from the uterine cavity or vagina. In catarrhal or idiopathic variety of leucorrhea, the discharge is in mild and liquid forrn but does not excoriate or irritale the parts. But, when it is dependant inflammation organic lesions of uterus or its appendages the discharged becomes fetid, corrogive, acrid, browish or green.
- The discharge from the uterus is often from uterine cavity, more albuminous, thick, viscid, flocculant, and has an allkaline reaction, whereas vaginal discharge is always acidic, thin, white, creamy and milky.
- Leucorrhoeal discharge is more profuse and copious at the time of menses than at any other time but in some ladies, it continuously goes on, though quantity of discharge varies.

Effects of Leucorrhoea

- If the discharge is copious and continues for a much longer period, there could be heaviness in the epigastriurn and pain. There is also capricious hunger, nausea and vomiting, fainting spells, desire for those things which have no relation to the malady; digestion is difficult and slow; vertigo, headache; slow motion and general lathargy, pain particularly in shoulder-blades and generally in all the limbs; face is pale, livid, skin is discoloured and dull.

• When the leucorrhoeal discharge continues for a fairly long period, the patient feels exhausted even on any attempt to slight exertion. She grows weak and then, palpitation and breathlessness, dull and vacant looks, margin of eyes surrounded by black rings, all intellectual faculties are weakened, face is bloated.

Causes of Leucorrhoea

• Affects mostly nervous, lymphatic, feeble, cachetic ladies who have fair complexion, pale skin and soft skin.

• No age is immune from its attack-it can occur anytime between 15-45, though even children at the fairly much yonger age (say 8-10) have been the sufferers.

• There is hardly any endemic leucorrhoea, though undoubtedly some regional foods ae deficient in certain elements whic trigger episode of leucorrhoea.

• Depression, self mortification, brooding, chagrin, sudden shocking news or death, loss etc.

• Eating oysters, crabs, fish, acid fruits, hard water, beer, cider, too much use of tea, coffee, purgatives.

• Self-vice or onanism, too much indulgence in sex act, nymphomania, presence of foreign bodies within vagina (like pessaries, sponges etc.)

• Menstrual irregularitis, vaginitis, uterine displacements, pregnancy, miscarriage, worms in intestines, confinement, easy-going life style, pulmonary pthisis, chronic consti-pation.

• Piles, diarrhoea, suppression of sweat, milky secretion, bronchial expectoration, vomiting, cold in the head.

- Cancers and ulcerations, local inflammations engorgement of cervix (neck of the uterus).
- Presence of gonorrhoea, resulting in inflammation, chancres, other growths.

Leucorrhoea of recent origin is not, at all, difficult to cure but, when in chronic form, treatment is not only difficult but much tedious also, as one has to cure not only leucorrhoea but also other concommittant symptions.Complications accompanying this disease are most difficult to cure than the main disease itself.

Leucorrhoea Treatment

- Take shivallingi (a root) and grind and sieve it. Have 5 gms. of this powder everyday with milk as the first thing in the morning for the desired result.
- Grind 10 gms. of turmeric and boil it in 100 gms. of water. When cold, wash the private part at least thrice a day with this water. Besides this take a batasha, put about 8 to 10 drops of the milk of a Banyan and swallow it daily before sunrise for about a week. Druing this time the ladies should avoid physical contact with their husbands. Even otherwise they should observe continence and lead an ascetic's life till they are fully cured. Any physical contact, in such condition might infect their husband's body too.
- The dried and powdered bark of the Mulsari (mimusops Elengi) tree mixed with an equal weight of raw sugar should be taken in nine grams dose every morning with water. Alternatively, equal weights of the leaf shoots of Bastard Teak (Dhak) and Banyan tree should be dried and powdered. An equal quantity of raw sugar should be mixed with them and nine gram doses should be taken with 250 ml. milk thrice daily. The root of the silk cotton tree is another specific herb for this condition. Seven grams of its powder with an equal weight of raw sugar should be taken with a glass of milk. Or, dry

amla and liquorice in equal quantities and powdered and mixed with thrice the quantity of honey make an effective drug against the disease. Six grams of the linctus should be taken in the morning and evening with milk.

Regimen: A strict dietary regimen is needed: fried foods and spices, pickles and savouries should be avoided. The patient should take betelnut after meals as it has curative effect. Late night and sexual inter course are of course taboo during the course of disease.

■

Heart Problems and High Blood Pressure

Though, during heart disease one should consult a heart specialist. Here some common home and ayurvedic medicines are prescribed for the knowledge of the readers.

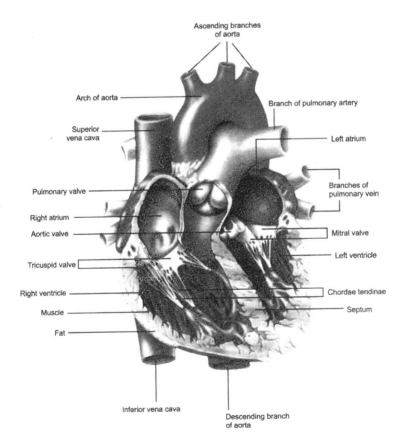

Ascending branches of aorta

Arch of aorta

Branch of pulmonary artery

Superior vena cava

Left atrium

Pulmonary valve

Branches of pulmonary vein

Right atrium

Aortic valve

Mitral valve

Tricuspid valve

Left ventricle

Right ventricle

Chordae tendinae

Muscle

Septum

Fat

Inferior vena cava

Descending branch of aorta

HYPERTENSION

In now a days fast moving life, the patients of high blood pressure are increasing day by day. To check hypertension, we should manage our life style.

- The patient should reduce as much as taking salt. He should have easily digestible food minus spicy condiments.

- He should have as much water as possible. Sometimes it is due to the malfuncioning of kidneys. Lot of water intake will help curing the basic defect.

- He should avoid taking tea, cigrettes, coffee and rich creamy biscuits.

- He should try to do light exercise and resort to massage of the body if possible.

- Have as much fruits as possible instead of regular food.

- The patient should try to keep his bowels clean. Constipation adds to the impurities in the body and thus put extra load on the expulsion system of the body.

- Drink curry leaves (curry patta) juice initially 3 times a day (1 glassful) for 1-2 months and then reduce to only once in the morning. Have it on empty stomach. For taking out juice, fill your mixer with washed curry leaves, add 1/2 - 3/4 glass water. Churn well and sieve. Add 1/2-1 lemon juice and drink fresh.

- A few cloves of garlic if taken on an empty stomach not only corrects the condition known as flatulence, but also lowers high blood pressure.

- The best remedy for hypertension is, sarpagandha (Rauwolfia Serpentina, which has been used in India for many years to deal with nervous disorders like insanity and high blood pressure. Alkaloids of this drug which have a direct effect on hypertension have been isolated and are being widely used by the practitioners of modern medicine, but they have certain unpleasant side effects which the drug taken in raw form does not have. Practitioners of Indian systems of medicine have therefore, preferred to use the root of the drug in a powdered form. Half a teaspoonful of this drug taken thrice a day deals with hypertension effectively.

- Drink coriander (dhania) juice made from fresh dhania (same way as curry leaves juices) 3 times a day. If this is not effective, start, having fenugreek (methi) juice instead (made from fresh methi) and if this is also not effective, move to curry leaves juice. Drink each juice for 10-12 days at least before you decide. If it is not working then move to the next one.

LOW BLOOD PRESSURE

- Have juice of basil (tulsi) leaves (10-15) mixed 1 teaspoon honey.
- Add 3/4 cup crushed liquorice (Mulathi) root to 4 cups cold water and allow it to stand for 2 hours. Then bring it quickly to a boil and steep for 5 minutes. Add this to the bathwater in the tub.
- Brandy or Alcohol of any variety in quantity from 15 to 50 ml. diluted with warm water, is a temporary expedient which can be tried till the exact cause of the malady is ascertained. Or, spirit of Ammonia Aroma should be given in teaspoonful doses diluted with an equal amount of water.

Giddiness Due To Blood Pressure

- Soak 1 teaspoon each of powdered amla, coriander seeds (saboot dhania) and sandalwood in a cup of water overnight. Strain and drink the next day. Continue for a few days.

High Cholesterol

- Sunflower seeds contain a substantial amount of linoelic acid which is helpful in reducing cholesterol deposits on the walls of the arteries.
- Finely dice an onion and mix it with 1 cup buttermilk along with 1/4 teaspoon black pepper (kali mirch) powder and drink.
- Regularly intake garlic (lahasun) cloves for a few days.
- Regularly intake coriander (dhania) decoction made by boiling 2 teaspoons dry coriander seeds (dhania) powder in 1 cup water. (milk and sugar can be added to impove its taste. This could be a welcome substitute for teas or coffee.)

Colourless Nails

Nails are the mirror of one's health. Their getting disfigured or colourless or brittle is a sure indication of something being wrong in the system. Normally the lack of calcium and vitamin D in body is usually manifest through the nails. Since beetroot supplies these nutrients, such persons must consume beetroot as much as they can both as salad and as vegetable. In winters if after eating beetroots one cares to sit in the sun, Vitamin 'D's deficiency shall be made good soon.

Insomnia

- Give to patient just one leaf of tulsi for chewing it and spread rest of the leaves evenly below his pillow and the corners of bed below the bedsheet. As the smell of tulsi leaves strikes his nostril, the person will feel sleepy and soon he will fall into sleep.
- Fry cumin seeds in a little ghee and grind to a powder. A teaspoon of fried powder of cumin seeds (jeera) mixed with the pulp of a ripe banana should be taken at night regularly.

- 2 teaspoons juice of fenugreek (methi) leaves alongwith 1 teaspoon honey may be taken daily.
- Soak 1 tablespoon leaves of fresh mint (pudina) in 1 cup of water for 30 minutes. Drink it every night. (do not boil).
- Take seeds of watermelon and white poppy seeds (khuskhus) and grind them separately. Mix equal amount by weight. Have 3/4 teaspoon once in the morning and once before sleeping. Take for 1-3 weeks as needed.
- Have raw onion with meals particularly with dinner.
- Consume plenty of curd. Also massage head with curd before washing. This is very helpful.
- Add 2 teaspoons of honey to a big cupful of water and have it before going to bed. Babies generally fall asleep after having honey.
- A cup of warm milk sweetened with honey should be taken before going to bed. Have it everyday.
- Juice of celery leaves (ajwain ka patta) with thick ribs and brittle stalks mixed with a tablespoon of honey when had at night before retiring helps to relax into a restful sleep.

Angina Pectoris

- Thoroughly mix 2 teaspoons almond oil with 1 teaspoon rose oil. Rub gently on the chest, morning and evening.
- Boil 1 teaspoon fenugreek seeds (methi daana) in 1/2 cup of water. Strain and add 2 teaspoons honey. Take twice daily.

HEART ATTACK

- Take 1/2 teaspoon garlic (lahasun) powder everyday.

Heart Burn

- Add 1 tablespoon mint (pudina) leaves to 1 cup water. Take twice or thrice a day.

Heart Pain
- Boil 1/2 teaspoon sandalwood powder in 1 cup water. Drink thrice daily.

Heart Palpitation
- Boil 1/4 teaspoon powdered cardamom (chhoti illaichi) seeds in tea water and drink.

Heart Weakness
- Regular intake of ripe bananas strengthens the heart.

Heart Troubles
- Tulsi is very effective to cure all sort of heart troubles. Since it controls blood pressure and keeps blood clean, its regular consumption prevents heart attacks. For special tonic for heart, prepare the medicine in the following way. Take about 1 gm. dried powder of tulsi leaves, add 3 gms. of the powder of Arjun tree and mix even amount of honey. Now either churn or mix them till the solution is fully homogeneous. Take about 1 gm. of this paste, add a little more of honey and lick it at least thrice a day, preferable early in the morning as the first thing an hour after lunch and as the last thing before your retiring for the day.
- Eat 1/4 teaspoon asafoetida (hing) along with one large raisin (munakka) everyday.

Tachycardia (Palpitation)
- Concoction of sevati (rosa alba) flowers, preserve of apple or carrots, in a dose of ten grams in silver foil should be eaten daily for some days. Or, carrots may be buried in hot ashes: when tender they should be taken out sliced and placed in open overnight in a ceramic dish to catch the dew. In the morning they should be sprinkled with sugar and rose water and eaten for some days regularly. Equal weights of

aniseed, dry coriander and jaggery (gur) should be powdered and taken in six grams doses after each meal. Five grams of aniseed. Three of coriander and 11 pieces of raisins should be steeped in water or rose water overnight and strained in the morning before drinking.

Anaemia

Anaemia or the lack of red blood corpuscles and haemoglobins is called Pandurog in Ayurveda. It may be caused by loss of blood through excessive menstruation, injury or any other cause in which excessive bleeding takes place, or due to defective blood formation because of injections, toxins and drugs or the inadequate intake of iron.

- Since beetroot is rich in iron it helps in enhancing the quantity of blood in the system. If one takes adequate amount of chukandar (beetroot) in salad or as vegetable this trouble gets cured in about a month. Having lemon juice drenched beetroot pieces as the first thing in morning is an ideal way of checking out the blood in body. Especially the ladies must consume beetroot in this manner during their periods.

- Soak 10-12 currants (munakkas) in water overnight. Remove seeds and eat them. Have for 2-4 weeks.

- Have spinach juice of 125 gm. spinach everyday, for 2-3 weeks.

- Foods rich in iron, honey, almonds, bananas, apricot (khumani), raisins (kishmish), fenugreek or salad leaves, onion, spinach (paalak), grapes, tomatoes, carrots, gooseberry (amla), beetroots (chukander), apples, pomegranate (anaar). Have plenty of them if you are anaemic.

- Carrot is a very rich source of iron and if taken raw with a few pieces of chukander (beetroot) it is certain to remove this trouble. Have fresh carrots and beetroot, liberally sprinkled over with lemon juice and munch your way to pink state of health. Vitamin 'A' and 'C' would not only keep your body strong but your blood red without any impurity. This is the surest cure of anaemia.

- Mix 1 tablespoon amla juice mashed with a ripe banana and eat 2-3 times a day.
- Have a ripe banana with 1 tablespoon honey, 1-2 times a day.
- Take freshly prepared apple juice an hour before meals or just before retiring for the night. For proper absorption of the juice, remember the stomach should be relatively empty when you have juice and also do not take anything for about half an hour after the juice.
- Avoid drinking tea and coffee immediately after meals as the tannin present in these interferes in the absorption of iron from food.

Blood Deficiency
- Take 2 teaspoons of amla juice and mix it with two teaspoonfuls each of honey and lime. Add 1 teacup water and drink on an empty stomach every morning. Whenever fresh fruits are not available, dried amla can be used. Soak 1 tablespoon the previous night in a cup of water. (Note: The treatment should continue for at least 120 days to achieve expected results.)
- Mix 1 tablespoon juice of amla with a ripe mashed banana and eat twice or thrice a day.
- Soak 2 or 3 dried figs (anjeer) in 1 tea cup water. Eat them along with milk next morning for a month.

Giddiness
- Soak cumin seeds (jeera) in lime juice overnight. Keep this mixture under the sun till completely dry. Bottle it. Chew 1/2 teaspoon of this mixture and drink with a glass of warm water.

(18)

Miscellaneous Disorders

ABSCESSES

An abscess is an enclosed pocket in the tisue filled with pus, usually caused by the body's reaction to bacterial infection.

Symptoms

Abscesses are accompanied by heat, pain, swelling, redness, and tenderness over the site of the abscess. Fever may be present, but not always. Abscesses are difficult to heal without treatment.

Complications

Sometimes abscesses must be surgically drained in order to release the pus. If the abscess is severely painful, or if you observe any red streaks radiating from the area, get immediate medical attention.

Homoeopathic Medicines

☞ Hepar sulphuris and Silica are the most common medicines for abscesses.

☞ For an abscess that is exquisitely sensitive to pain, cold, and touch, in a very irritable chilly person, give Hepar sulphuris.

☞ For an abscess from a foreign body give Silica unless the symptoms are particularly like Hepar sulphuris.

☞ For abscesses that are purplish or mottled, left-sided, and much better from discharging, in a talkative, intense person, give Lachesis.

☞ For abscesses that are very foul-smelling in a chilly, sweaty person with bad breath and a bad or metallic taste in the mouth, give Mercurius.

Self Care and Home Remedies

☞ If the abscess is draining, cover it with a gauze dressing and keep the area clean.

☞ Alternating hot (five minutes) and cold (one minute) wet compresses stimulates circulation and healing.

☞ Use massage techniques of specifically promote drainage of the lymph system.

☞ A combination of echinacea and goldenseal (two dropperfuls of tincture in water three times a day or two capsules four times a day) can be useful to stimulate the immune system to fight infection.

☞ Apply Calendula tincture (diluted one part to three parts water) to the area once it has drained.

☞ Give betacartotene: 50,000 IU once a day.

☞ Give zinc: 30 mg once a day.

☞ Give vitamin C: 1000 mg two times a day.

BLEEDING

Bleeding, or hemorrhage, is a flow of blood from the arteries, veins, or capillaries, occurring internally or through any of the natural openings of the body or from damage to the tissues or blood vessels. There are many causes of abnormal bleeding, ranging from wounds, trauma, and acute conditions, such as a nosebleed, to chronic conditions such as hemorrhoids, hemorrhagic disorders, or cancer.

Symptoms

Bleeding is characterized by a flow of blood, ranging in colour from bright red to black, from anywhere in the body. The blood may spurt if it comes from an artery, or flow more passively if it originates in a vein. The most common symptoms of blood loss are weakness, fatigue, dizziness, a faint feeling, thirst, perspiration, and, later, changes in pulse and breathing. Anemia is confirmed through a complete blood count.

Complications

Extreme blood loss due to injury, postpartum hemorrhage (after childbirth), uncontrolled uterine bleeding due to other causes or undetected internal bleeding can result in anemia, dehydration, shock, or death. Get medical attention immediately if blood loss is severe.

Homoeopathic Medicines

☞ The first medicine to give for bleeding resulting from injury or trauma is Arnica.

☞ For bleeding in which the person has bright red cheeks, consider Belladonna or Ferrum metallicum.

☞ For blood loss in a weak, pale, collapsed person, give China.

☞ If there is dark blood oozing from various parts of the body, give Crotalus horridus.

☞ For bleeding from the veins with a full feeling in the veins, the medicine is Hamamelis. If the bleeding is caused by a fall or overexertion and the blood is bright red, look at Millefolium.

☞ For a person who bleeds easily and the blood is fluid, bright red, and without clots, give phosphorus.

Self Care and Home Remedies

☞ Take whatever first-aid measures are necessary to stop the bleeding, including applying pressure directly to the injury with a clean cloth or by applying pressure to the pressure points above the injured area or by wrapping the injury with gauze or cloth.

☞ Apply Calendula tincture or a combination of Calendula and Hypericum tinctures directly to the bleeding area.

☞ Never apply topical Arnica preparations to open wounds because they can cause a rash.

☞ Dried cinnamon applied directly to the area can sometimes stop bleeding.

☞ Geranium, Trillium can all be taken internally for bleeding. Take one half teaspoon of tincture every one to two hours up to four times a day.

If weakness occurs from bleeding, take iron supplementation. The dosage depends on the form of iron, the degree of anemia and the cause and degree of bleeding.

BRUISES

Bruises are caused by trauma that doesn't break the skin, resulting in blood leakage into the tissues.

Symptoms

Black and blue or purplish green discoloration under the skin with sore, aching, pain.

Complications

Discoloration may take a long time to go away. The area can remain tender.

Homoeopathic Medicines

☞ Arnica is the first medicine to think for any bruise.

☞ Give Bellis perennis for bruises to the veins or from leakage from the veins after blood drawing or for ordinary bruises if Arnica fails.

☞ Give Ledum if the bruise is cold and feels better from cold.

☞ Give Ruta for bruises on the outer covering of bones (periosteum), such as on the shins.

☞ If the bruising tendency is chronic or recurrent, Phosphorus may work.

☞ Think of Sulphuric acid if Arnica doesn't work after injuries.

Self Care and Home Remedies

☞ Ice a bruise right away to keep more blood from leaking out into the tissues.

☞ Wrap an Ace bandage around the area, not too tightly, to support the area and control the extent of the bruise.

☞ After twelve hours, alternating hot and cold moist packs can help healing and remove discoloration.

☞ If a person is susceptible to bruising, bioflavonoids (1000 mg per day) strengthen the veins.

BURNS

Burns are caused by heat, electricity, radiation, hot water, or particular chemicals. The skin may be inflamed, blistered (second degree), or charred (third degree). The most common burns are sunburn and burns from fire or touching something hot.

Symptoms

First degree: redness, heat, swelling, and pain.

Second degree: all of the above plus blistering and oozing.

Third-degree: significant charring of tissues.

Complications

Burns can be serious, even fatal, depending on the extent of the body that is burned and the degree of the burn. Any extensive burn-even first degree should receive medical attention. First degree burns will heal without extensive treatment in most cases. Palliative treatment will help relieve pain and inflammation. Second and third degree burns may cause scarring and infection. Third-degree burns can be life threatening if extensive and may require treatment in a hospital setting. Get medical attention immediately for a third degree burn.

Chemicals will continue to burn the skin as long as they are present; wash them off immediately with lots of water. Get medical attention for serious electrical burns.

Homoeopathic Medicines

☞ The first medicine to consider in most burns is Cantharis.

☞ For scalds, either give Cantharis first, then Urtica urens if there is not improvement within theirty minutes, or, if the other symptoms fit Urtica urens, give it first.

☞ For chemical burns, the after effects of old burns or burns that are slow to heal give Causticum.

☞ For electrical burns, give phosphorus.

Self Care and Home Remedies

☞ Soak the burned part in cold water or ice water, or apply cold wet compresses to relieve pain and inflammation. Calendula or Hypericum tincture may be added to the water as described next.

☞ Apply Calendula spray, gel or tincture, diluted one part tincture to three parts water. Dilute more if the tinctue hurts to apply. Hypericum tincture may be used, diluted 1:3 as well. On first degree burns, Calendula gel or salve may be applied. Calendula tincture, diluted one part Calendula to three parts water, can be very useful in first and second degree burns.

CHICKEN POX

Chicken pox is an acute viral disease, usually in young children, associated with the varicella zoster virus, which also causes shingles. It is spread by infected droplets from the nose or throat.

Symptoms

A period of mild headche, fever, and general discomfort followed by numerous fluid-filled sores, which crust over. Once crusts form, the contagious period is over. Normally once a person has chicken pox he will never get it again.

Complications

Chicken pox is very contagious and may cause scarring. The sores may become infected. Do not give aspirin to a child with chicken pox, because they may get Reye's syndrome—a type of brain and liver illness characterised by nausea and vomiting and a sudden change in mental functioning with lethargy, loss of memory, and disorientation, leading to coma.

Homoeopathic Medicines

☞ The most common medicine for a very itchy chicken pox is Rhus toxicodendron.

☞ If the sores ooze a honey like discharge and scab over, and the tongue is coated white, think of Antimonium crudum.

☞ If the main symptom is a loose, rattling cough, take a look at Antimonium tartaricum.

☞ For out-of the ordinary fussiness in a child who doesn't want to be touched or looked at, consider Croton tiglium, especially if the skin feels very tight.

☞ If the child is very clingy, weepy, and thirstless, look at Pulsatilla.

Self Care and Home Remedies

☞ Oatmeal bath: use Aveno (avoid the type that contains camphor) or place one cup of finely blended dry oatmeal in the bath to soothe the itching.

☞ To treat infected sores, apply a few drops of one part Calendula tincture diluted with three parts water and cover with bandages or gauze.

CUTS, SCRAPES, AND PUNCTURE WOUNDS

A wound is caused by a sharp object piercing the skin. It may be a cut (laceration or incision), a puncture wound, or a scrape (abrasion).

Symptoms

Tissue damage, bleeding, bruising, inflammation, swelling, and pain are the most prominent symptoms of wounds. the seriousness of the wound depends on the amount of damage to underlying organs and tissues.

Complications

Superficial wounds are not serious, and usually heal rapidly on their own if they are kept clean free of infection. Deep cuts may need stitches. If cuts or puncture wounds are deep, damage to organs, muscles, nerves and bones needs to be assessed immediately by a qualified medical practitioner. A sserious wound, such as a knife or gunshot wound, may be life threatening.

Puncture wounds carry the risk of tetanus within two days to two months after a wound has been infected. Deep or dirty puncture wounds should have dirt and dead tissue removed by a qualified medical practitioner to help prevent tetanus. Early signs of tetanus include jaw stiffness, difficulty swallowing and stiffness of the neck, arms, or legs after a wound. More advanced tetanus includes the inability to open the jaw (lockjaw), a fixed smile, and raised eyebrows, as well as spasms in the neck, back and abdomen. Tetanus may be fatal if untreated. If the person has not had a tetanus immunization or booster in the last five years, a tetanus inoculation should be given immediately following the injury.

A dose of homoeopathic Ledum may be given immediately as well.

Homoeopathic Medicines

☞ The first medicines to consider for puncture wounds are Ledum and Hypericum.

☞ If the affected part is cold and cold to the touch, give Ledum.

☞ If there is numbness or shooting pains, use Hypericum.

☞ If there is bruising or bleeding, give Arnica.

Self Care and Home Remedies

☞ For serious wounds: Apply direct pressure to stop bleeding. Get medical attention immediately.

☞ For minor wounds: Apply direct pressure to stop bleeding. Clean the wound with soap and water.

☞ Apply Calendula gel, cream, or spray (for abrasions), or tincture, diluted one part tincture to three parts water. Dilute more if the tincture hurts when applied. Calendula prevents and heals infections. Hypericum tincture may be used, diluted one to three parts as well, especially for infected cuts or scrapes. Use the tinctures several times a day until there is definite healing, then once a day until healing is complete.

☞ Cover the wound with a bandage or gauze dressing.

☞ Change the dressing as needed.

☞ For minor puncture wounds: Clean the wound with soap and water.

Let the wound bleed freely to flush out diret or debris unless bleeding is severe.

☞ For severe bleeding: Apply direct pressure on the wound. Soak puncture wounds in warm water several times a day to remove more debris.

☞ Apply full strength or diluted Calendula tincture to promote healing.

☞ For general wound healing: Vitamin C (500 mg four times a day).

☞ Zinc (30 mg per day).

☞ Beta-carotene (50,000 IU per day).

INSECT BITES AND STINGS

Everyone has had the experience of a bee sting or an insect bite. It is usually just annoying, painful, or inconvenient, putting a damper on a perfect outing or picnic. Sometimes it can cause a severe allergic reaction or anaphylactic shock.

Symptoms

Redness, swelling and itching occur after the bite, sometimes with burning or stinging pain. Hives, difficult breathing, and shock may occur with severe anaphylactic reactions. Signs of anaphylactic shock are paleness, perspiration, confusion or unconsciousness, rapid pulse and shallow, irregular breathing.

Complications

Occasionally the person who is bitten or stung can have a severe allergic or anaphylactic reaction, which can be life threatening. This may occur from a second bite or sting when there was not much reaction to the first one. Get medical attention immediately if the bite is from a poisonous insect or spider, or if there is difficutly in breathing, severe swelling, or loss of consciousness. Consult a physician if you think the person may have been exposed to Lyme disease; a red circle resembling a target around the site of a deer tick bite is one early symptom. Antibiotics may be necessary to avoid later complications of heart and muscle or joint disease.

Homoeopathic Medicines

☞ The first medicine to give if there is swelling is Apis.

☞ For bee stings, give Apis.

☞ For bites with terrific itching, consider Caladium.

☞ In the case of anaphylactic shock, call ambulance and give Carbolic acid or Apis.

☞ For most insect bites, first try Ledum.

☞ For wasp stings, Vespa is the first choice. Use Apis if Vespa is not available.

Self Care and Home Remedies

☞ Remove the stinger with a flicking motion using a fingernail or a sterilised needle. Pulling it straight out may release additional venom.

☞ Apply an ice pack or a cold, moist pack to reduce swelling and circulation, and to prevent the spread of the venom.

☞ Clense the area with soap and water.

☞ Calendula (Marigold flower) cream can ease itching and irritation.

MEASLES

Measles is a viral disease that affects children and adults who do not have active immunity. It is highly contagious and is spread by airborne droplets from an infected person before the rash apears and during the first few days of the disease.

Symptoms

Fever (up to 104°F), runny nose, sore throat, cough, sensitivity to light, and an extensive pink to brownish pink, irregular, itchy rash starting around the ears, face, and neck which then lightens up as it spreads to the trunk and limbs as the fever decreases. Koplik spots, which appear only in measles, look like tiny grains of sand with a red ring and are usually seen opposite the first and second upper molars on the inside of the cheek.

Complications

Secondary infections with streptococci and other bacteria may occur causing pneumonia, ear infections, and other infections. In one out of a thousand children, measles can cause encephalitis with fever, convulsions, and coma.

Homoeopathic Medicines

☞ Give Aconite if the symptoms come on suddenly and violently with a high fever, especially after a fright or exposure to cold dry wind.

☞ Euphrasia is used for measles when there is a lot of sensitivity to light and a discharge from the eyes.

☞ Gelsemium is the medicine when measles comes on more slowly and the child is dizzy, drowsy, droopy and dull with a fever and headache in the back of the head.

☞ Pulsatilla is used in the later stages of measles when thick yellow green discharge and a low fever are present and the rash is beginning to fade.

☞ Sulphur is used when the rash is late to develop, and is purplish or dusky and the itching is made worse by heat and bathing.

Self Care and Home Remedies

☞ Bed rest in a darkened room.

☞ Drink plenty of fluids.

☞ Eat a light diet, depending on appetite.

☞ Vitamin C: 250 mg twice a day for young children, 500 mg two times a day for adults.

☞ Keep sores clean and avoid scratching them.

☞ Apply cold compresses to the sores.

MOTION SICKNESS

Motion sickness, also known as sea, air, or carsickness, is a complex of symptoms caused by stimulation of the balance mechanism in the inner ear by repeated motion. Disorientation, without being able to see a fixed horizon during motion, can induce motion sickness. It can be compounded by emotional stress.

Symptoms

Nausea and vomiting are the primary symptoms. Salivation, sweating, paleness, and hyperventilation are also common. Mental confusion can also be present.

Complications

Dehydration and lack of eating can produce problems if the motion sickness is prolonged.

Homoeopathic Medicines

☞ Cocculus is the most common medicine for motion sickness.

☞ Petroleum is good for the combination of motion sickness and skin problems.

☞ Sepia is useful for motion sickness that is complicated by hormonal problems or relieved by vigorous exercise.

☞ Tabacum should be used when motion sickness is extemely severe.

Self Care and Home Remedies

☞ Try to sit in the place in the vehicle where there is the least motion. Stare at a fixed point for orientation, not at anything that is moving.

☞ Lying down or reclining may help.

☞ Look above the horizon at a forty five degree angle.

☞ Get some fresh air.

☞ Eat small amounts of food frequently.

☞ Eat Saltime crackers to help relieve the nausea.

☞ Eat bland foods such as broth, rice, and pasta.

☞ Tea and toast are usually well tolerated.

☞ Sip ginger root tea to help relieve nausea.

☞ Stimulate Stomach an acupressure point in the soft place below the knee and to the outside of the leg where the tibia and fibula bones meet. Use firm rotary pressure on the spot for a few seconds. Repeat when needed.

SUNSTROKE, HEATSTROKE AND HEAT EXHAUSTION

These are conditions resulting from oversensitivity or prolonged exposure to the heat or the sun.

Symptoms

Heatstroke, also called sunstroke, is a reaction to exposure to the sun which often begins with a headache, dizziness, and fatigue leading to heat, flushig, and dryness of the skin. Perspiration is usually, but not always, decreased. The pulse rate increases quickly, sometimes up to 180 beats per minute, and breathing rate often increases also. The person can become disoriented and unconscious, as well as having seizures. Body temperature can shoot up very quickly to 104°F or even 106°F.

Heat exhaustion, which is less severe, is characterised by gradual weakness, nausea, profuse perspiration, anxiety, and fainting. The skin is generally pale and clammy. The pulse is weak and the blood pressure is low. Notice that the primary differences between the two are perspiration and the pulse.

Complications

In heatstroke, collapse of the heart can lead to permanent brain damage or death. Heat exhaustion is usually temporary and rarely has complications. If the body temperature is rising rapidly and the person has the symptoms of heatstroke /sunstroke, seek emergency medical attention.

Homoeopathic Medicines

☞ Belladonna and Glonoine have very similar indications for this condition. Unless the main complaint is a bursting or exploding sensation in the head, give Belladonna first.

☞ If there is no improvement within fifteen minutes, or if there are other clear symptoms that point to Glonoine, give Glonoine.

Self Care and Home Remedies

For heatstroke: Take immediate measures to cool yourself by taking a cold shower or bath, or wrapping yourself in cold towels or ice.

For heat exhaustion: Lie with the head down. Replace fluids and salt.

HAY FEVER

Hay fever, or acute allergic rhinitis, is a reaction to pollens from grasses, trees, and flowers. Bouts of hay fever often occur annually when pollens are released, generally in the spring, summer, or fall.

Symptoms

Runny nose with clear watery discharge, sneezing and itchy eyes, nose, and mouth are the common symptoms. Headache and irritability often accompany hay fever. People who have it often feel miserable. Many hay fever sufferers also have allergies at other times of the year.

Homoeopathic Medicines

☞ The most common medicine for hay fever with watery eyes, watery nasal discharge and sneezing is Allium cepa.

☞ If there is an irritating discharge from the nose and a bland discharge from the eyes, consider Allium cepa.

☞ If itching of the nose and palate is the primary symptom, give Arundo or Wyethia.

☞ When eye symptoms, especially watering are the most significant symptoms, give Euphrasia.

☞ When the eye discharge is irritating but the nasal discharge is bland, give Euphrasia.

☞ When the discharge is like egg white and the person has cold sores or canker sores, a headache, and perhaps a recent disappointment, rejection, or grief, Natrum muriaticum is the medicine.

☞ If sneezing is the most prominent symptom, strongly consider Sabadilla.

Self Care and Home Remedies

☞ Use an indoor air purifier to remove pollens from the air.

☞ Vaccum your living and work areas more often during hay fever season.

☞ Bioflavonoids can be helpful.

☞ Some people find nettles to be of benefit, either in tes, capsule, or tincture form.

☞ Take 500 mg of Vitamin C twice a day.

FEVER

Fever is a symptom, not a disease in itself. The body raises its temperature in order to fight infection when the immune system is in the process of responding to foreign invaders such as bacteria and viruses.

Symptoms

When your body temperature rises over 100°F, you have a fever. Fever is a beneficial reaction of the body to illness, and as such should be allowed to run its course unless it is very high. Chills often precede or accompany fever, and sweats occur when the fever is going down or "breaking." Fever may occur in the absence of infection, and in some cases it may be of unknown origin.

Complications

☞ Fever rarely goes above 105°F, but it may induce febrile seizures at that point. A high fever with a severely stiff neck may be caused by meningitis, a life-threatening disease that requires immediate medical attention. Homoeopathy is quite effective in dealing with the bacterial or viral infections that cause fever, even in cases in which antibiotics have failed. However, in serious infections with high fevers that do not respond to homoeopathy, medical attention should be sought.

Homoeopathic Medicines

☞ Use Aconite or Belladonna for fevers that come on suddenly and violently.

☞ Fevers that need Aconite often start after a shock or fright or exposure to a cold dry wind.

☞ Belladonna is useful when the fever is high, the person's face is red, and the fever is accompanied by a throbbing headache.

☞ When the fever is intermittent or comes at the same time every day, consider China.

☞ Give Ferrum phosphoricum for fevers in the first stage of illness with few other symptoms than red cheeks.

Self Care and Home Remedies

☞ If fever is high, sponge you forehead, palms, soles and may be complete body for half on hour. Then cover up the body.

☞ Drink plenty of water.

☞ Sage, basil or ginger tea may be of some help if cough accompanies fever.

■

How to Take
Homoeopathic Medicines

Homoeopathic medicines should be taken on the basis of symptom-similarity.

Start from the 30 potency, if you are taking medicines in liquid form for acute problems.

If the problem is chronic then start with 200 potency, once in a day or sometimes once in a week (as directed by your physician)

Sometimes a higher potency is required and that is used once in ten days as for example 1000 (1 m) potency and that too in early morning, empty stomach.

For acute conditions when you are using 30 potency, take three to four drops in one fourth cup of water, three to four times a day.

When you are using biochemic medicines, use 6x potency and take four tablets three times a day.

In case of children the dose should be half of the adult dose.

In case of any confusion, you can write to me on Palm-11/03, Shipra Sun City, Indrapuram, Ghaziabad, U.P. or consult an educated and experienced homoeopathic physician.

Use only sealed medicines and that too of reputed companies like WSI, SBL, Ralson, Bioforce, Bakson, Beck and Koll, Reckweg etc.

20

Methods of Preparation of Gharelu Nuskhe

Powder: Dry material in shade. Crush to make fine powder and sieve through a cloth.

Paste: Powder the materials, heat with a little water and make into fine paste or crush the material, add a little water and grind to make a paste.

Fresh Juice: Wash the material (parts of Plant) and remove dirt. Chop the plant into small pieces and crush well. Squeeze the crushed material through a cloth and collect juice.

Decoction: Wash the material (Dry of Fresh) to remove the dirt. Chop into small pieces. Boil ½ cup of material in four cups of water and reduce into one cup. Filter the decoction and use.

Milk Decoction: Wash the material and make it into small pieces and pound it. Boil half cup of it with one cup of milk and four cups of water. Reduce it to one cup. Filter it and use.

The ratio of ingredients is given in each column separately. It should be taken preferably in empty stomach. Any food should be taken only after one hour of taking decoction (Kashaya).

Instructions: Generally all the preparations are for internal use. In other cases special description is given on how to use (external, gargle etc.). When honey, milk, hot water, jaggery, sugar etc. are mentioned as vehicle, it should be taken in sufficient quantity. If the course of medicine is not mentioned it has to be taken till there is relief for the complaint.

Triphala is a group of three fruits namely Haritaki (Harad), Vibhitaki (Baheda), Aamalaki (Aamla), Trikatu consists of three pungents called Pippali, Marich, Sunthi (Dry ginger).

The above mentioned medicines can be used at a primary health care level and also as preventives. Most of these conditions need very systematic treatment. So please get the advice of a good physician for specific, severe and prolonged illness.

■

21

Biochemic Combinations
for Children

There are 28 combination compounds of biochemic remedies which are detailed hereunder with main symptoms for which each one should be used. These combinations are numerically numbered.

Before purchasing any biochemic combinations, make sure that only products of standard homoeo companies are purchased (e.g. WSI, SBL, Ralson, Bakson, Bioforce etc.)

BIOCHEMIC COMPOUNDS

Number-1	Anaemia
Number-2	Asthma
Number-3	Colic
Number-4	Constipation
Number-5	Coryza
Number-6	Cough, Cold and Catarrh
Number-7	Diabetes
Number-8	Diarrhoea
Number-9	Dysentery
Number-10	Enlarged Tonsils
Number-11	Fever
Number-12	Headache
Number-13	Leucorrhoea
Number-14	Measles
Number-15	Menstruation Troubles
Number-16	Nervous Exhaustion

Number-17	Piles
Number-18	Pyorrhoea
Number-19	Rheumatism
Number-20	Skin Diseases
Number-21	Teething troubles of Children
Number-22	Scrofula
Number-23	Toothache
Number-24	Tonic for Nerves and Brain
Number-25	Acidity, Flatulence and Indigestion
Number-26	Easy Dilivery/Parturition
Number-27	Lack of Vitality
Number-28	General Tonic

Dosage for children and adults have been mentioned on each combination but in emergent situations like cholera, diarrhoea, colic, flatulence, fever etc dosage may be repeated with greater frequency but quantity of dose will, however, remain the same. In case of any confusion or difficulty a Homoeopthic physician should be consulted.

MOSTLY USED BIOCHEMIC COMBINATION NO. 21 (TEETHING TROUBLES)

These tablets help to build up general health of the baby and also keep him free from most of the health problems which normally occur during dentition period. It is a combination of Ferrum Phos and Calcarea Phos which in combined form, proves more effective and efficacious due to addition of Ferrum Phos. Mothers generally prefer to use Calcarea Phos but, in my view, this combination should be preferred in comparison to single use of Calcarea Phos. If these tablets are used regularly (from the anticipated time of cutting teeth) until your child can be relieved from the agony of dentition problems.

22

Home Treatment by Turmeric (Haldi)

Haldi is stringent and sour in taste. It is a time-tested beauty aid and a nourishing herb which not only gives natural gloss, royal glow and lustre but also imparts vigour an dyouthful vitality to the entire body. Haldi is thus a great tonic in general, aromatic, diuretic, expectorant, blood-purifier, skin-tonic, carminative, pain reliever, germicidal, anti-flatulent, producer and enhancer of red blood corpuscles, anti-phlegm. atic, antibilleous, protector of eyes, anti-inflammatory and imparts coolness to the system.

Bruises, sprain and wounds

(i) Applying past of Haldi powder with lime or water on the effected part-eliminates swelling and pain in bruises.

(ii) Taking 1 teaspoon. Haldi powder with hot milk is also useful.

(iii) Filling the wound or cut, (from which blood is coming out) with haldi powder-will stop bleeding and curing of the wound/cut.

(iv) Applying poultice made of gram flour, Haldi powder mixed with mustard or til oil-on the sprained portion-enhances blood circulation and gives relief.

(v) Tying a bandage of haldi (prepared with 4 teaspoon flour, 2 teaspoon haldi powder, 1 teaspoon, pure ghee, ½ teaspoon sendha namak with water) on the bruised portion gives relief.

(vi) Giving fomentation with cloth soaked in hot water (500 gm. water boiled with 1 teaspoon sendha namak and 1 teaspoon haldi powder) on the bruised part eliminates pain and swelling.

(vii) Giving fomentation with Potli (having one ground onion mixed with 1 teaspoon haldi powder) heated with yil oil on the bruised portion gives relief.

(viii) Applying haldi powder heated in ghee or oil on the wound and tying it with a bandage helps in quick healing of the wound.

(ix) Dusting haldi powder on wounds also helps.

Skin-problems

(i) Ringworm white spots applying paste of haldi rubbed on stone with water on the effected portion is useful.

(ii) **Skin eruptions**—Applying paste of Haldi and till oil on the body prevents skin eruptions.

(iii) Applying haldi powder or paste on the body before bath is a preventive against skin problems and also a depilatory. (clears the growth of hair on body).

(iv) Urticaria:

    (a) Taking 1 teaspoon haldi powder with 1 teaspoon mishri or honey twice a day cures urticaria.

    (b) Taking halwa (made from 2 teaspoon flour, 1 teaspoon ghee, 1 teaspoon haldi, 2 teaspoon sugar, 1 cup of water) in the morning cures Utricaria.

(v) Tiking roasted haldi with gur cures itching.

(vi) **Eczema:** Sucking tablet of ground haldi with honey for 10-15 days cures Eczema.

(vii) **Pustules:** Placing cotton dipped in Haldi oil over pustules gives relief.

(viii) **Freckles, spots:** (a) Applying Haldi rubbed on stone with water eliminates them. (b) Massaging the face with

Ubtan (mix ground Haldi with milk of banyan or pipal and soak it overnight) 1 hour before bath eliminates freckles on the face and imparts natural glow.

Cough and Cold, Asthma

(i)   Taking haldi powder and little salt with hot water or sucking a small piece of haldi or licking 1 teaspoon haldi powder with ¼ teaspoon honey-gives relief in 4 cough and eliminates congestion of bronchi.

(ii) Taking ¼ teaspoon haldi with hot milk is helpful in checking running nose.

(iii) Inhaling the smoke of burnt haldi throws out the trapped phlegm.

(iv) Taking ¼ teaspoon powder of haldi (roasted in hot sand and then ground) with hot water relieves.

Breathing Problem (Asthma)

(v)   Taking Haldi boiled in milk and sweetened with Jaggery is very useful in cold and Asthma.

(vi)   Sucking a piece of haldi (like lemon drops) or keeping it in mouth at night cures chronic cold.

(vii) Licking tablets (made by mixing haldi powder, barley powder and bansa-ash in equal proportion and honey and making small tablets) 4-5 times In a day eliminates trapped phlegm in the body.

(viii) Massaging the throat and chest with little haldi powder, ground black peppio mixed with ghee-cures irritation in bronchial chords.

(ix)   Giving a pinch of haldi powder with milk to children gives quick relief.

(x)   Inhaling smoke of cow-dung cake with haldi sprinkled on it, releases the trapped phlegm.

(xi)   Taking ¼ teaspoon of haldi powder with 3-4 gulps of warm water-acts as a preventive against attack of Asthma.

Whooping Cough

(i)   Taking 1 teaspoon ground roasted haldi powder wfth two spoons of honey 3 or 4 times a day gives relief in cough.

(ii) Taking Pan with little haldi piece in it is also useful.

Indigestion and Stomach Problems

(i)   Taking haldi powder and salt in equal quantity with warm water gives instant relief in acidity.

(ii) Taking 1 teaspoon churna (grind haldi 4 gm., Sonth 4 gm., Black pepper 2 gm. and ilayachi 2 gm.) after meals is digestive, eliminates wind and stomach ailments.

(iii) Taking curd or whey with haldi powder after lunch cures digestive problems.

Sore-Throat

Licking Haldi powder mixed with honey 2-3 times a day cures soreness.

Tonsilitis

Fomentation with paste made of 10 gm. haldi powder roasted in mustard oil and then tied around the neck gives relief in Tonsils.

Blisters in Mouth

Gargling with 1 glass of water in which little haldi powder is boiled, twice a day, cures it.

Urinary Troubles

Taking paste of ground or juice of raw Haldi and honey with goat's milk (if available) twice a day, cures all urinary problems.

Small-pox

(i)   Taking 1 teaspoon powder of haldi and imli (tamarind) for 4-5 days acts as a preventive against small-pox.

(ii)   Applying a thin layer of the ubtan (haldi powder, foam of fresh milk and wheat flour mixed with mustard oil or fresh cream) on the affected part twice a day-flattens the deep spots of Small-pox and makes the skin soft.

Worms

Licking the paste (made of ¼ teaspoon haldi powder and ½ teaspoon Vayavidang choorna with 1 teaspoon of honey for 7-8 days kills worms and throws them out.

Pregnancy and Postnatal Care

(i)   Taking 5-10 gms. of HaIdi powder with water-during menses is an antipregnancy dose for ladies.

(ii)   Taking 1 teaspoon with hot milk in latter part of the 9th month of pregnancy helps in easy delivery.

(iii)   Taking 1 teaspoon roasted haldi powder with gur after delivery eliminates weakness and cures uterus swelling.

Pain in Breasts

Applying paste of haldi rubbed on stone on the affected part eliminates pain.

Gout

Taking laddu of haldi (mix ½ kg. roasted ground haldi, one finely grated dried Coconut 1 kg. jaggery, 200 gm. cashew nuts or ground nuts and make laddu) daily in the morning with Tulsi or lemon tea-makes the joints supple and gives relief in pain and swelling.

Pain in Ribs

(i)   Applying paste of haldi powder mixed in hot water-on the aching ribs gives relief or

(ii)   Massaging the ribs with haldi oil or

(iii) Massaging the ribs with paste of Haldi powder in milk of the Aak plant gives quick relief.

Jaundice and Liver Problems

Taking 4-5 gms. of haldi powder mixed in a glass of whey twice a day activates the liver.

Diabetes

Taking 4-5 gms. ground haldi with water or honey twice a day is helpful in curing diabetes.

Leucorrhoea

(i) Taking haldi powder with sugar twice a day for sometime checks this.

(ii) Washing the private parts with haldi water (10 gm. Hhaldi boiled in 100 gm. water) is also useful. Alongwith it taking one batasha with 8-10 drops of milk of banyan tree before sunrise for 7 days helps in early cure.

Debility in Males

Taking about 7-8 gms. of raw ground Haldi and equal amount of honey with goat's milk cures debility in males.

Dental Problems

(i) Rinsing the mouth with haldi water (Boil 5 gms. Haldi powder, 2 clove and 2 dried leaves of Guava in 200 gms. water) gives instant relief.

(ii) Applying and rubbing the teeth with paste of haldi powder, salt and mustard oil-strengthens the gums.

(iii) Massaging the aching teeth with roasted ground heldi eliminates pain and swelling.

(iv) Keeping piece of roasted haldi near the aching tooth and letting the saliva ooze out also helps.

(v) Filling the cavity in teeth with roasted ground haldi powder gives relief from pain.

(vi) Applying the powder of burnt haldi piece and ajwain on teeth and cleaning them makes the gums and teeth strong.

Ear troubles

Putting one or two drops of haldi (by roasting 2 pieces of haldi in mustard oil) in the ear, cleaning it with an ear-bud cures ear-problems.

Eye-troubles

(i) Cloth dipped in the solution of Haldi powder and,water is employed as an eye-shade.

(ii) Dropping haldi water (1 teaspoon haldi powder boiled in 500 gms. water till 125 gm. water is left. Cool and strain it through a fine cloth) in the eyes twice a day and putting the cotton soaked in water on the eyelids relieves pain, redness, irritation and itching in the eyes.

(iii) Applying, bit heated paste of piece of haldi rubbed on stone on eyelids also eliminates pain, swelling and eye-troubles.

(iv) A decoction of haldi powder with water as a cooling lotion on the eyes is useful in conjunctivities.

Poison of Insect-bite

Applying the mixture of Haldi powder and lime over the affected part nullifies the toxic effect.

Coryza

Inhalations of fumes of burning haldi passed into the nostrils relieves coryza.

■

Home Treatment by Basil (Tulsi)

It is one of the most sacred plants of India. It has many medicinal hot properties.

CATARACT

Extract the juice of Tulsi and add a little of honey to it. Apply this over the eye every morning and evening. If the cataract be of raw type, it shall be cut away and if it be of ripe type, it shall be ripened soon to enabel the doctor to remove it by operation.

COLD AND COUGH

The chronic patient of this problem have their hair going untimely white. To stop the process and cure it, take 300 gms. of Tulsi leaves dried in shade, 50 gms. of Dalchini, 100 gms. Tejpata, 200 gms. sonff (aniseeds), 200 gms. of small cardamom, agiya 300 gms; Banfshaw 25 gms; red sandal 200 gms. and Brahmi herb 200 gms—grind all these ingredients and strain them through a cloth. Now take 10 gms. of this powder, boil it in 500 gms. water and when just a cup of this water remains, add sugar and milk and drink it twice a day like you have tea. All these problems will vanish in a couple of days.

DIRTY WATER-PURIFYING AGENT

Sometimes people don't like water of a new place. Just put a couple of Tulsi leaves and then you'd face no problem. If you put just two leaves of Tulsi in a pitcher of water for an hour or so, and then remove them, the water shall be purified immediately.

EAR-PAIN

Take about 10 leaves of Makoy and the leaves of Tulsi. Extract their juice together and put it in the affected ear when it is slightly lukewarm (heat it a little in the Sun). Alternatively add half a tablet of Camphor in Tulsi juice and put this juice in the ear for instant relief.

EYE TROUBLES

Put a drop of Tulsi juice mixed with even quantity of honey for all sort of eye troubles, especially pain and burning. This solution can also be preserved in a bottle. If there be the problem of trachoma, grind ten leaves of Tulsi together with a clove. Put it into your eyes every four hours. If there be swelling in the eyes, add a little of Tulsi-juice with alum and apply in your eyes for instant relief.

EPILEPSY

Rub Tulsi juice over your body every day after taking your bath. Keep the blossoms of Tulsi inside the fold of your hanky every tiem. At the time of attack, smell the blossom deeply. Should the attack make one unconscious, grind 11 leaves of Tulsi, add a little salt to it and put a few drops of this juice in the patient's nostriles. He would immediately regain his consciousness. Keep a Tulsi plant in your varanda or somewhere near your bed room.

FLATULENCE

Take about 10 gms. of Tulsi juice, 10 gms; of dry ginger and 20 gms. of jaggery. Mix all of them together to form small tablets. Take this tablet thrice a day with water to set right your digestive process. But during the period you have this trouble, better keep fast or take only easily digestible food.

FISTULA

Have three or four Tulsi leaves every morning with water. Alternatively take the root of Tulsi plant and the fruit of Neem tree (Nimboli) and grind them together. Take 2 gms. of this combination every morning with whey for quick relief.

FLU

Take about 10 gms. of Tulsi-leaves and 250 gms. of water. Boil them together till water is halved. Now add in the remaining water rock salt, according to taste. No sooner did you start to sweat that the effect of flu shall be removed with the sweat and you shall be alright. Alternatively drink Karha of Tulsi leaves, black pepper and batasha for still quicker relief.

HOARSE VOICE

Just extract the juice of 10 Tulsi leaves, add a little of honey and lick it. Just a small spoonful quantity of this solution will soothen your throat nerves and your voice will be again sweet.

HAIR TROUBLE

Put about 21 leaves of Tulsi and 10 gms. of Anwala Churna in a big bowl. Add a little of water to make a paste of them. Apply it evenly on your head and allow it to dry. Then wash it with cold water. This will prevent hair loss and clear dandruff also.

HEART TROUBLES

Tulsi is very effective to cure all sort of heart troubles. Since it controls blood presure and keeps blood clean, its regular consumption prevents heart attacks. For especial tonic for heart, prepare the medicine in the following way. Take about 1 gm. dried powder of Arjun tree and mix even amount of honey. Now either churn or mix them till the solution is fully homogeous. Take about 1 gm. of this paste, add a little more of honey and lick it at least thrice a day, preferably early in the morning as the first thing, an hour after lunch and as the last thing before your retiring for the day.

HYSTERIA

If the hysteric effect be due to excess of phlegm in the body, make the patient smell Tulsi leaves and drink 5 Tulsi leaves juice. If it is caused by the excessive heat going to the head, grind five Tulsi leaves and five black pepper by mixing them in water and make the patient drink this water every morning and evening for a week's time. They hysteria will be cured.

INDIGESTION

Take the seeds of Tulsi and peepal in equal quantity and grind them to fine powder form. Now add 3 gms. of this powder with a spoonful of honey and lick it twice a day to clear indigestion.

Drinking the tea of Tulsi leaves also brings quick relief. The filthy substance will get out of the body with sweat and urine. Alternatively add 1 gm. of rock salt in 10 gms. of Tulsi leaves' paste and swallow it down with water.

INSOMNIA

The easiest and best treatment of this problem is to pluck 51 leaves of Tulsi. Give to patient just one leave for chewing it and spread rest of the leaves evenly below his pillow and the corners of bed below the bed sheet. As the smell of Tulsi leaves strikes his nostril, the pereson will feel sleepy and soon he will fall into sleep.

ITCHING

Extract juice of Tulsi and massage on the parts of the body itching. If the trouble be chronic, take about 2 parts of Tulsi juice and one part of til oil. Allow them to parboil on slow fire. Then cool it and put it in a bottle. This is a most effective oil for all sorts of itching problems.

JAUNDICE

Add 10 gms. Tulsi-leaves' juice in about 50 gms. of radish juice. Add a little of jaggery to the combination to sweeten it. Have this solution twice or thrice daily for about a month for getting total relief from this problem.

Alternatively take 3 gms. of Tulsi-leaves' juice and 3 gms. of the root of Punarnava. Mix them both in 50 gms. of water and drink it for about 15 days. This is a very effective dose to cure Jaundice.

KIDNEY TROUBLES

For any type of kidney trouble, Tulsi-juice provides a very effective cure. Just soak 5 to 7 gms. of Tulsi seeds overnight in water. In the morning grind them with sugar and drink the combination. Soon the congestion or infection in kidney will be thrown out by means of copious discharge of urine.

LEPROSY

Living in an atmosphere abounding with Tulsi plant is the best treatment. For white patches chew 5 leaves of Tulsi every morning, evening and afternoon. Licking the combination of Tulsi leaves' juice with honey will cure the trouble quickly.

LEUCODERMA

(i) Add a few drops of lime-juice in Tulsi-leaves' juice; (ii) grind 10 gms. Tulsi-leaves with a clove of garlic and apply the paste on the affected portion every day, 10 days for total relief.

LETHARGY

The tea made of tulsi-leaves provides instant energy and makes one quite energetic. This is not a cumbersome preposition because as you prepare tea, so you prepare this Tulsi tea and instead of putting tea-leaves, put Tulsi leaves.

The regular intake of this tea shall not only provide energy but will also keep you away from all the diseases borne out of the vitiation of kaph (phlegm) in the body.

MIGRAINE

Get a small bunch of Tulsi blossom; dry it in the shade and grind it to powder form. Just take two gms. of it, mix about half a spoonful of honey to it and make the person lick it. God willing, you may never require second dose, for it is a very efficacious treatment. In case you feel like, have another dose by the evening for a total cure.

MOUTH-BOILS

Take just a leaf of Chameli plant, and four leaves of Tulsi. Chew them properly for a few minutes and suck in the juice. In about a day the trouble will vanish.

MALARIA

Take about 10 gms. of Tulsi leaves' juice and add to it 1 gm. of ground black pepper. Administer this dose five or six days after every two hours. Alternatively make small tablets of this combination and feed the patient on Tulsi tea additionally. In a couple of days the fever will vanish alongwith the malarial infection.

NIGHT BLINDNESS

Put two drops of Tulsi leaves every morning and evening and drink the juice also at three times a day. Continue the treatment for about a month time for total cure.

Black pepper is also very effective to cure this trouble. Put some black peppers' grain in a wet cloth to allow them to bloat up. Now remove their rinds and grind them in Tulsi juice. Line this paste in your eyes every morning and evening for total cure.

NOSE-BLEEDING

The easiest and most effective cure of this trouble is to keep the Tulsi blossom near you and smell it as and when you like. For those who are chronic patient of this trouble, this simple treatment is very effective and cures the trouble almost totally. Drinking Tulsi juice mixed with honey will also help and provide extra strength to the body.

PARALYSIS

Boil a few leaves of Tulsi in a tumblerful of water. When cool, strain and put this water in a bottle. Massage this water on the affected limbs. Continue this treatment for at least two weeks. This treatment, coupled with regular intake of the Tulsi leaves will produce the desired results.

PNEUMONIA

Get the pure Tulsi oil from a recognised Ayurvedic medicine shop. Put this oil on the chest of the afflicted person. Together with this treatment, extract the juice of five Tulsi leaves, mix with it a few ground grains of black pepper at 6 hourly interval. This combined treatment will produce enough heat in the body to make the person sweat. With sweat all the effect of cold inside the body shall vanish and the patient will be cured.

CHICKEN POX

If the person be already afflicted with this problem, then giving Tulsi leaves' juice mixed with Ajwain (Bishop's seeds) will provide relief. But to prevent this menace afflicting you or your family members, prepare anti small pox tablets in the following way and administer one tablet daily with water.

Take 5 gms. Tulsi leaves, 2.5 gms. Javitri,1/2 gm. real pearl ash, 20 grains black pepper, 1/2 gm. saffron and 1/4 gm. cloves. Add Ganga water to make these tablets.

SPLEEN ENLARGEMENT

Take 5 gms. Tulsi leaves dried under shade, 5 gms. Indra Jau and grind both of them to powder form. Add a little of salt and take the combination with a glass of cold water. Continue this treatment every morning and evening for 10 to 15 days. The effect of Tulsi leaves will bring spleen to size and cure the trouble.

SLUGGISH LIVER

Take 5 Tulsi-leaves, 2 gms. roasted powder of cumin seeds' and 2 gms. of black salt. Grind them together to make it come in a homogeneous powder form. Add to it even amount of the kernal of the wood-apple. Mix the combination in about 100 gms. of curd to reactivate the sluggish liver. For early relief from any sort of stomach disorder, drink a spoonful of the combination of the juices of the tulsi and ginger.

STONES

Make the patient sit on a chair having a commod like opening on the seat. Now prepare the Karha of the blossoms of Tulsi, i.e., boil about 100 gms. of Tulsi blossom in a kilo of water. When the vapours start emerging, bring the container and stove beneath the chair on which the patient is seated. The moment the vapour starts touching the private organ, it would dissolve the stone. Continue this treatment for about a week for total cure.

T.B.

Grind together 5 grains of black pepper and five leaves of Tulsi leaves. Then mix the combination with half a spoonful of honey and lick it. Make the patient lick this combination twice daily. If it be winter season, add a little of ginger juice, the husk of wheat and a little of salt also in the combination. This is a very effective treatment but it has to continue quite long. Externally, rubbing a little of Tulsi juice and ginger juice's mixture over the lungs shall bring the desired relief. Continue the treatment for about two months. Continue antitubercular treatment too.

TESTES PROBLEM

If there be swelling on the testes or any other problem concerning with testes, apply the paste prepared in the following manner over the testes. Take about 5 gms. each of a camel's dung. Amarbel (easily available in Mango groves), the leaves of Arhar and Tulsi-leaves. Grind them to a homogeneous paste in a little of cow's urine. When the paste is ready, apply it over the testes thickly. Allow it to dry and remove it in the morning. A week's treatment will cure all troubles connected with the testes.

URINARY PROBLEMS

For any sort of this trouble, soak about 5 to 7 gms. of Tulsi seeds overnight in water. In the morning grind these seeds in water, add a litttle of sugar to the combination to make it more tasty. Drink this combination early in the morning and also in the afternoon, i.e., twice a day. Soon you will have copious discharge of urine and all problems connected with the urinary tract shall vanish in a week's time. Continue drinking raw milk and water mixture at least twice a day also.

VENEREAL DISEASES (MALE)

Tulsi leaves juice is very effective to cure all sort of these troubles. Take 5 gms. each of Tulsi seeds or dried Tulsi leaves and 5 gms. of tamarind. Now adding a little of honey to the combination make small tablets. These astringent tasting tablets should be taken at least four times a day. Don't swallow these tablets but suck it slowly.

If the accompanying cough be of dry type add a little of honey then additionally, make the patient have the combined juice extracted from the even amount of Tulsi seeds, ginger and onion. In case of wet-cough add sugarcandy also in the combination.

WORMS IN EARS

If an insect be gone inside the ear of if there be worms in the ear or ears, in either case dropping a few drops of lukewarm Tulsi juice will provide immediate relief. If there be swelling in the ears, then add the juice of Bhangra with the juice of black Tulsi and put a few drops of this juice inside the affected or both the ears for quick relief.

ACIDITY

Take the dried blossom of Tulsi, rind of the Neem tree, black-peppar and peepal in even quantity and grind them to powder form. Take 3 gms. of this powder every morning and evening with plain water. All the acidic effect of the body shall pass out with urine and sweat. But remember, never to take milk over Tulsi leaves which might afflict your skin.

BLACK SPOTS

These are caused by excessive indulgence in the sexual pleasures which sap your vitality and these black spots appear. Extract a little of juice of Tulsi and add two times more lime juice. Make their homogeneous solution and apply this solution or paste over these spots every night with soft hands. The spots will be removed in a week's time. But restrain your sexual urges.

■

24

Home Treatment
by Fruits and Vegetables

ACIDITY

The easiest and tried and tested remedy to cure acidity to have as much cucumber or kakadies as one can without sprinkling salt over it. For if you sprinkle salt over them, you again use something which adds to the acidity. After you have eaten your normal meal, don't drink water over it but have kakadis or cucumber. You can also have them with your food also.

ANAEMIA

There are many fruits and flowers which offer permanent cure for the patient:

(i)   Give the patient half a kg. of sweet grapes' juice for 10 days. He shall have enough blood in the body with rich haemoglobin in it.

(ii) Have (Peaches) Aaddoos at least 5 at a time—for about 10 days. Aaddoos are rich in iron and they would cure this trouble.

(iii) Suck about 200 gms. of Falsey every day. If you like you can chew them also.

(iv) Have mango-juice and milk combination for about a week.

BALDNESS

Take the oil of the mango pickle and massage your skull for about half an hour with it. If you are bald not because of the hereditary effect, you would definitely get back your hair. During the season of kakadis (cucumber) crush them and extract their juice and apply it on your hair for a fortnight. You can also apply their pulp on your head for quick hair-growth.

BED WETTING

Feed such children on dry dates (Chuhare) pieces before they go to sleep. Don't let them have tea when it is dark. Give them Halwa of potatoes instead. The most effective treatment for such chronic patients is to give them about 2 gms. of the powdered stone of Jamun with water. In a couple of days this problem will be solved for ever.

BLOOD IMPURITY

Shahtoot has this admirable quality to cure all the impurities of blood. Just take about 250 gms. of Shahtoot early in the morning instead of your normal breakfast and follow it up by the even quantity of Shahtoot in the evening also. These two doses will cure the blood totally.

BRONCHITIS

Take about 10 almonds and 10 dried raisins (Munnakka) and soak them in water overnight. Early in the morning remove the rinds from Badam (almonds) and unseed the raisins. Now take a small, cleaned piece of ginger and grind the three ingredients to a paste form. Now add two spoons of honey and lick it. Do it every evening and morning for two days. This treatment will not only cure the trouble but would also strengthen your lungs.

BURNING IN URETHRA

First, try to ascertain the cause of this burning. If it is caused by the unhygienic condition of the area, clean it by lukewarm water. If it is caused by eating lots of chillies, stop eating them. Always drink a lot of water half an hour after having your meals. If it is being caused by some inside problem, extract the juice of the fresh Anwala, add a little of sugar candy and drink it thrice a day. In just three days' time this trouble will be cured. Anwala will cleanse the renal region which is causing the burning and then this problem shall be over. But always keep the area clean.

CHOLERA

First of all extract the juice of a couple of onions and give it to the patient. Then prepare the lemon syrup and ask the afflicted person to drink it slowly by gradually sipping it. If still the patient be feeling nausea, then feed him again on the onion juice. Add a little of lemon juice and black-pepper, rock salt also in the onion juice. This dose will definitely cure the trouble. But keep on making the patient drink lots of water. O.R.S. powder is available an every medical store, which can be of great help in curing cholera.

CONSTIPATION

(i)   Take about two spoonfuls of gulkand and drink a glass of lukewarm milk in the night, over it. Next day you will have clear motion.

(ii) Have mangoes and then drink a glass of hot water over it for curing the trouble.

(iii) Have half a cup of peaches juice for quick cure of the constipation.

(iv) Howsoever chronic be your constipation, if you take a glass of diluted orange juice on empty stomach after brushing your teeth, you'll never have this problem.

Cough: If the cough be of dry type (having no expectoration of phlegm), then take the kernal of the mango-stone, reduce it to powdered form and lick the it at least twice or thrice every day till fully cured.

In case the cough be with phlegm expectoration, take the rind of a pomegranate and keep on licking it. Alternatively, extract the juice of ripe apples and drink at least half a glass of it every morning and evening for complete cure. Having ginger and boril leaves and boril leaves juice mixed with honey shall also help.

CHRONIC WOUND

Bring a piece of mango bark and boil it in water to make its thick paste. When the paste cools down a bit, apply daily on the wound. This paste is anti-septic and full of healing qualities. The best way to apply it is to take it on a soft cloth or cotton, put it over the wound. Do it every evening and morning. In three or four applications the wound would heal up. If the would be quite deep, it might take longer time for the new flesh to appear. Keep the would clean by washing it with warm water. In homoeopathy a drug colemdula is made from Genda flowers, which is a great antiseptic.

DIABETES

Extract half a cup of Jamun juice and add equal amount of Karela juice. Mix them drink and the mixed juice as the first thing in the morning. In about a fortnight the miraculous effect can be seen. Together with it, grind the stone of Jamun to powder form and keep it in a clean bottle. Take this powder daily—only half a spoonful—every morning and evening with water. These remedies shall not only help cure diabetes but will also help check the onset of diabetes. In about three months time the total relief could be expected.

DYSENTERY

Take about 10 gms. each of the kernal of jamun and mango stones and grind them to powdered form. Mix about 2 gms. of this mixture of the powder in 100 gms. of curd and eat it. Do so at least twice a day, preferably after breakfast and lunch. In summers you can also take it during the night. This regular intake will cure the trouble in about a week's time. But such persons must not ocnsume fried and fat -rich items and should start taking a long walk in the morning.

DRUG INTOXICATION

If the person is having Bhang or opium intoxication, then treat the afflicted person in the following way:

(i) Ask the patient to take a Guava and allow him to sleep. The intoxication will be cured.

(ii) If it is not be guava season, you can have a few soft leaves (1015) of guava, grind them and extract their juice. Give it to the patient for drinking.

(iii) To kill the heat of the intoxication, extract a little juice of tamarind and give it to the person for drinking. This will quickly cure the intoxication.

(iv) Ask the patient to sick the Lemon. This is also helpful in curing bad effects of intoxication.

ECZEMA

Normally we throw away the thick covering of the water-melon (Tarbooz). If we burn it and keep the ash in a clean bottle, this is a very effective remedy for eczema. If eczema be of weeping type, just sprinkle a little of this ash for quick relief. If it be for dry type, add this ash to a little of mustard oil and apply it on the affected part. In about a week's time the skin will become soft and healthy. But don't touch tea or coffee for about a week.

EAR-BOIL

Collect a little of green blossom of mango normally lying beneath the mango tree. Extract the juice of this green blossom, add in even amount of mustard oil and put a few dr   in the afflicted ear. This treatment will make the boil burst and clear out all the pus etc.

EARLY AGING

Take about 10 almonds, soak them in water, remove their rinds and grind them to paste form mixing a little of milk. Now boil the combination in milk and when cool, add about two spoonfuls of honey. Drink this portion like you are sucking it. Continue the treatment for about a year. Have lots of apples, grapes and oranges daily.

EXTREME THIRST

Normally the thirst is easily quenched by drinking juices of orange, pineapple or caneapple. Still if you fail to quench the thirst then try the following remedy:

Take out the kernal from a mango-stone and crust it and boil it in water like you boil tea. Now add a little of sugar candy and drink it like you drink tea.

For those who frequently feel extremely thirsty, pomegranate juice mixed with sugarcandy is the ideal combination. Drink it twice or thrice to overcome this feeling.

EPILEPTIC ATTACK

For those affiliated with epilepsy, phosphorus rich fruits are essential. If they continue to have the juice of Shahtoot (25 gms. only) daily, this divine juice will provide enough strength to the nerves to fight out this affliction. In the absence of Shahtoot, the juice of ripe apples or Sev Ka Murabba (Jam of Apple) should be given. Figs also help the nerves to acquire strength. Lightly roast figs on fire and allow the patient to eat it, and wash it down with the juice of ripe apples.

FIRE BURNS

If the fire-burn be not very deep, extract the kernal from the mango stone, rub it against water—wet surface and apply the rubbed paste on the burns. Soon the cool relief will be felt. If it be a form of wound, burn the dry leaves of mango, strain the ash and sprinkle over the wound. This ash is antiseptic and very good to heal the fire burns.

FATIGUE

Narial-Pani (coconut-water) immediately removes fatigue and brings energy back to the body. Having orange juice with little of pineapples juice mixed in it shall quickly remove the fatigue. While drinking these, rinse them in your mouth and keep you tongue standing clean of the teeth for quick rejuvenation.

FOUL SMELL FROM BREATH

Normally this foul breath is caused by not any infection in the mouth but due to digestive disorders. Take five grains of Munnakka (raisins) and five pieces of small cardamom. Remove the seeds of Munnakka and replace them by the grains of small cardamom. Lick their juice without chewing them. Soon your breath would become fresh.

GOUT

Get the oil from the kernal of mango stone extracted and then use this oil in massaging the aching joints. This massage cures even the most chronic aching joints. Alernatively, have 125 gms. of 'Chaman Ka Angoor' (the grapes from CHAMAN), regularly in your breakfast for at least a fortnight for getting total relief from the trouble. Then after reduce the quantity of the grapes dose and enhance the intervening period. Grapes do not allow any raw phlegm to settle on joints.

GIDDINESS

Take 10 Munnakkas (raisins) and immerse them in a glassful of water. Keep the glass in such a position that solar rays strike direct at the portion of glass containing Munnakkas. This water heat will bloat up the Munnakkas. Now remove their seeds, chew the pulp of Munnakka and wash it down by the water Munnakkas were soaked in. The giddiness will vanish.

GONORROHOEA

Take about a handful of the seeds of musk-melon (Kharbooza). Remove their covering to get to their kernal. Now rub them against stone to grind them to make their Sherbat. Add about 10 drops of Sandalwood oil to it. Ask the patient to have twice this sherbat. Continue the treatment for about 10 to 15 days or till this illness is totally cured.

HAIR-LOSS

Sometimes malnutrition result in hair-loss. It means hair are not getting their due food and getting weak on their roots. Sometimes people who become habitual of Bhang or Afeem (opium) addicts suffer from this problem. The hair get too dry owing to malnutrition. Having Jamun and applying coconut oil externally is the tired and tested remedy to stop hair-loss. To regain hair at the skull, apply pulp of kakadi or kakadi (cucumber) juice-massage it and leave as it is for half an hour before bath.

HIGH B.P.

Cut a huge Tarbooz (water-melon) separate its seeds and sprinkle rock-salt and a little of black pepper. Do so while keeping it in a big steel plate. Now give all the cut pieces of the melon to your friends and relations and have only seeped out tarbooz -water is a very good tonic because it contains minerals like phosphorus iron and vitamins in rich quality. Those who can, may avoid salt at all or have very little of Sendha salt. This water is also a good tonic for nerves and nerves shall be relaxed also.

HEAT STROKE

The juice of raw mangoes popularly known as 'Panna' is a very effective anti-dote of heat stroke. Lightly roast a raw mango and crush it to extract its juice, throwing away the rind and stone. Now, in this juice add a little of black-pepper powder, common of rock salt and sugar. Just drink this juice and you shall not feel any adverse effect of heat. If one already is struck by heat, then applying pulp of tamarind over hand and feet will immediately lower the body temperature and the heat's effect will be neutralised.

HEART AILMENT

Juice of Mausambi is ideal to reduce the cholesterol level in the blood whose increase causes all sorts of heart ailments. Besides clearing the excessive cholesterol, Mausambi juice also brings freshness to the system. But drink this juice without ice as ice dilutes its effect. This juice would keep heart vessels soft and supple and blood with have smooth circulation also.

Alternatively mix sugarcandy powder in the even amount of Anwala-powder and have it every morning and evening with water for quick cure of all sorts of heart ailments.

INDIGESTION

Cut a fresh Papaya, sprinkle rock salt and black-pepper over its pieces and pour few-drops of lemon and eat them gradually. Papaya has a very useful element 'Pepsin' which is very good to clear any sort of indigestion. Not only it clears indigestion, but also cures the germs inside the body. It is an ideal fruit to activate the sluggish liver. Besides cleaning infection and curing indigestion, Papaya also provides energy to the body.

INFLUENZA

Take a Chakotara (botanical name Citrus Decumana) and cut it to small pieces. Then suck all these pieces one by one. Its juice is a very good antidote for the flu germs.

Alternatively, if a shaddock be not available, one can replace it by diluted orange juice. Extract the juice of 2-3 orange, add 1/4th water to it and sip this diluted juice twice or thrice a day. Having citrous fruits is helpful to cure flu because of the large quantity of Vitamin "C" in them.

IMPOTENCE

Take two Chuhares (Dried Dates) and 10 raisins—boil them and grind them together. Now add to it the ground paste of 10 almonds after soaking them overnight and removing their skin. Now add a little of honey in the paste and add both the pastes together. Now eat a spoonful or two with a glass of hot milk. Although it can be eaten with dinner also, yet in many cases this combination causes night discharge. Hence it is better to have this combination with breakfast. In less than two weeks the trouble will vanish.

JAUNDICE

Jaundice results when we eat infected food items. Here the colour of body becomes yellow. Hence such a patient must be fed on those fruits and flowers which have these contents in adequate quantity. Having Dates, Peaches, aloobukhara, whey from unsour curd, red raisin (Munnakka) beetorrt, tomatoes, strawberry mixed with honey will eke out these elements and you would again start to have your blood red and healthy. And jaundice shall automatically be taken care of.

KIDNEY PAIN

Having the decoction (porha) of the leaves of grapes quickly cures this trouble. Boil about 30 to 40 leaves of grapes in water, then add a little rock salt and strain it through a coarse cloth. Now allow the patient drink it. While preparing the Karha take care that you use only soft leaves and boil them after thoroughly cleaning them. This Karha is very effective to cure all sort of kidney troubles.

LIVER-TROUBLE

Tomato juice and soup of tomato is very effective to activate a sluggish liver. Make the patient drink the juice early in the morning and soup in lunch or dinner. For elderly persons juice of two tomatoes and for younger patient of one tomato would be adequate. Add a little of ginger juice with tomato juice to benefit the bowels also.

Alternatively collect the dried broken leaves of mango normally found lying beneath the mango tree, boil these the same way you boil tea-leaves and drink them like you drink tea just once a week to keep you liver in good working.

LICES

Take the rind of pomegranate, dry it and then grind it to put the dried powder in a bottle. Whenever any one has this trouble, add this powder in water to form a paste and apply this paste to hair. Keep it as it is and after half an hour of this application, wash it off. The lices will be cleared off the head. The powder of Sharifa seeds is also effective to clear lices.

LEUCORRHOEA

Those ladies who are afflicted with this trouble must take the powder of the kernal of mango at least twice or thrice a day with water. Another good treatment is having the starchy fluid of the rice mixed in Jamun juice. Another remedy is to hack of Katira Gond (gum) to small pieces, then soak them in water and have those bloated pieces of Gond with milk.

LOSS OF APPETITE

Many a time this loss of appetite results due to over-eating or eating very heavy food at irregular hour. In such a case, leaving food for a day or two is good proposition. If it is caused by some internal disturbances in the digestive system, then having 7 or 8 leeches would be best remedy. Do not eat them but gradually suck them. By the time you have licked the eight lichee your desire for food will increase. Having lemon-juice diluted in water is also very effective to restore your appetite.

MALARIA

This dreadful infection is caused by the mosquitoes. First of all you must keep your area clear of any filth and dirt. Since the fever comes after a shuddering sensation, the patient should be well covered in quilts or blankets. Give the patient diluted juice of shaddock to drink. Shaddock or Chakotara has the capacity to kill these germs.

Drinking Chirayata solution is an age-old anti-dote of malaria. To lessen its bitterness you can add a little of orange juice. Juice of cincona's bork is also useful.

MEMORY LOSS

Leechi and apples are very effective to revive one's memory cells. Have your normal food followed by a glass of whey seasoned with as afoetida and cumin seeds. Stop drinking water with your meals. With lunch drink a glass of whey and after dinner a glass of cow's milk having a little of honey mixed in it. If you eat a lot of leechies and apples, your memory would definitely be revived in about a month or so. Keep your system clear of constipation.

MISCARRIAGE

If there be no deficiency in the productive organs of the lady, then this problem can be successfully tackled with the help of the leaves of raspberry or Rasbhari. Such ladies, immediately after conception must drink the concoction of the leaves of raspberry. Prepare the concoction like you prepare tea. And instead of adding the leaves of tea, put the leaves of raspberry in the milk-sugar solution. These leaves are quite rich in iron, phosphorus and calcium which are the necessary elements to develop the foetus.

MOUTH BOILS

Take a few soft leaves of guava. Extract their juice, add a little cachet (Katha) powder and apply this paste over the mouth boils. Then allow the saliva to ooze out. Soon the boils would start drying up. Alternatively, add a well ripe banana in sweet curd. Now gradually apply this solution with the help of a spoon. A couple of doses of this dish will clean the mouth boils in a few days.

MIGRAINE

Those who have their houses located amidst the mango groves seldom suffer from this trouble. You must have seen parrots pecking up the mango blossom which lies scattered beneath the mango trees. Select a few bunches of green blossom and grind them to extract about half a spoonful of their juice. Put a few drops of this juice in the opposite nostril you are having pain in, or apply it by your finger. over your nostril. Now lie down in a dark room. In just a couple of days this problem shall be taken care of and you shall be cured.

NAUSEA

Take a bit of Aam Ka Papad and give it to the person suffering from this trouble. The feeling of nausea shall vanish soon.

Alternatively, if it be the mango season, ask the person to suck mangoes which has a very thin juice. If mangoes be not available, take about 25 gms. of orange juice and add about two spoonfuls of honey. Now make the afflicted person drink it drop by drop. Soon the feeling of nausea shall vanish.

NOSE BLEEDING

Extract the juice of green mango kernal by adding a little of water. Just two drops would be quite sufficient. Put these drops in each nostril to stop nose-bleeding. Look at a very good fruit and its consumption stops nose bleeding almost immediately.

NIGHT BLINDNESS

As we all know the night blindness is caused by the lack of Vitamin "A" in the system. Such persons should consume mangoes, tomatoes, cabbage and honey. The more of these items are consumed the better would be you eye-sight in nights.

NIGHT DISCHARGE

Add a little of alum in the juice of mango and apply this solution around your penis during sleep. Although it might give a sticky feeling yet in about 10 to 12 days you shall be rid of this problem.

To thicken your semen take about 2 gms. of Jamun-stone's powder mixed in about 5 gms. of amla powder with honey. Continue both the treatments simultaneously and you shall be totally cured of this trouble. But stop reading pornographic books or seeing dirty movies.

OBSTRUCTION IN THE URINARY PASSAGE

Just grind a few Anwalas and apply the paste on and around penis and the lower stomach. You would have copious discharge of urine. Cucumber or kheera is a very good diuretic agent. Hack off their tops, remove their skin and eat them as much as you like. Sprinkel a bit of common slat and lemon for better taste. Soon you will feel the urge to urinate and all the obstruction will pass out with it. You can eat a lot of musk—melon for this purpose. All these watery fruits are very effective diuretic agents.

PAIN IN KNEES

Strawberry is the ideal fruit to cure this trouble, since its chemical analysis revealed that after figs, the iron content is maximum in a strawberry fruit. It is equally rich in calcium. Have as much fresh strawberries as you like. You can always chew a few leaves of basil (Tulsi) for better result. Walking a lot and having strawberry are the necessary steps to cure this trouble permanently. Walk slowly but for a long distance.

PILES

For common type of Piles having the powdered form of the kernal of the mango-stones with whey is very effective. Take just 2.5 gms. of this powder with 100 gms. of whey. The haemorthoids will soon dry up. While continuing this treatment, smelling the blossom of mango will also help. For bleeding type, having Anwala powder with whey is good. The proportion should be 3 gms. of the powder and 100 gms. whey, Figs are also very effective. Soak about 5 figs at a time in water and have them in the morning and evening for early cure.

PARALYSIS

Although there could be innumerable reasons of paralysis, yet if it is caused by clotts in the brain or due to high blood pressure, the best is to feed the patient exclusively on apple, and grape juice. These juices are mixed in equal quantities and give to patients four time one up at a time. For external massage the best juice is that of a bottlegourd. Just extract this juice and rub it forcefully on the affected portion for relief. If it be winter season they dry fruits like almonds, casemnu and pista could also be included in his diet. If one strictly adheres to this treatment then in about two months ' time the cure can be possible.

PALPITATION OF HEART

If it be caused by some traumatic happening in the patient's life, washing of hands and feet will restore it to normal palpitation. If the cause be extreme heat, have just a couple of Leeches or Falsey or Aloobukhara. Soon the palpitation will be normal. If it is a chronic trouble then having juice of ground pomegranate leaves can provide quick relief consult your physician as soon as possible.

RICKET

Add equal amount of grape juice in orange and ask the patient to drink the lot at least three times a day. Just 50 gms. of juice at a time will do.

If the child be having teeth, then give him dates to eat after dipping them in honey. Just five to six dates with honey a day will be enough to make the child grow well in a week's time. If the child be just a infant, give him the syrup of honey to drink. Mix two spoonfuls of honey in a cupful of water to prepare this syrup. If the child be in the feeding stage, the mother should apply honey on her nipples before feeding her child.

SLEEP-WALKING

This is a very dangerous habit and can even prove fatal. In the modern life full of traffic any thing can happen to such a person. Such persons should be fed exclusively on mango and milk combination or what is known as 'Amar Kalpa'. During this period the person is not given anything else but mango and milk. Mango-milk combination would energise nerves to cure this trouble.

STONE IN BLADDER

Normally the seeds of grapes, oranges or munnakkas (raisins) are thrown away because they create stone. But if the seeds of grapes are crushed and their powder's only half gm. quantity is taken with milk every evening, stones will be dissolved and thrown out of the system.

The juice of pears is also capable to dissolve the stones. The juice of slightly raw type of apples is also effective to do so. But it should be taken with adequate quantity of black pepper sprinkled over it.

SWELLING IN SPLEEN

Jamun is very effective to cure all the afflictions connected with spleen. Drink the juice of Jamun every day in the afternoon for curing the swelling in spleen.

Alternatively, during the mango season drink a glass of mango-shake after adding a little of honey. continue this treatment for 21 days for total cure of this problem.

During the off-season of mango or Jamun, roast lightly a lemon and suck it after sprinkling rock salt and black pepper for about a week.

TONSILITIS

This is a very disturbing problem as the patient is unable to eat or drink properly. First of all, start the treatment by making the patient gargle with lukewarm water to which a little of alum has been added. After half an hour of this throat-cleaning process, drink half a glass of the juice of Shahtoot (cane-apple). The juice is not only antiseptic but also has admirable healing powers. Since its ultimate effect on the body is cool, it also lessens the pain in the throat due to burning. Continue the treatment for a couple of days for total cure.

TESTICLE SWELLING

Extract the kernal of the stones of leechi. Then lightly roast then over fire them grind them to paste form. Then apply it over the testicles while lukewarm. One or two applications will subside the swelling. If needed by you can repeat the remedy after a week or so.

Another very effective remedy is following: Take about two handfuls of mango leaves and add a little of salt to them. Now grind both of them. Add a little of water to make a thick paste, then heat it a little and apply over the testicles.

TEETH TROUBLES

(i) Collect the flowers of the pomegranate tree normally found lying beneath the tree. Dry them in the shade after cleaning them and then grind them to powdered form. Use this powder as tooth-powder. This is a very useful tooth-powder to stop blood oozing from the teeth, and also making teeth strong.

(ii) During the mango season, go to a mango grove early in the morning. Pluck a few of mango leaves, the soft ones —chew them repeatedly and then spit out the juice. Just in a week's time your teeth shall be firm and shining.

(iii) For those persons whose teeth have become disfigured because of eating too much of Pan Masala, etc. and have grown weak due to the effect of lime in the Pan Masala, the following tooth paste would be very good to keep the teeth firm and shining. Add a little of mustard oil in a spoonful of common salt and sprinkle a few drops of lemon juice over it. Daily rub your teeth with this paste to keep your teeth firm and sparking.

URINARY TROUBLES

If the urine be persistently having deep yellow colour, it means that the tract is infected. Add a little of plain sugar in the syrup of canebeerry (Shahtoot) and drink it at 6 hourly interval for two days. The infection will be totally cured.

In case you have the problem of repeated urination, take about five to six Lisore (cordial maxi tree's fruits, also known as Labhere and chew them repeatedly. Soon the repeated urination problem will cured. If Labhere be not available, take about 2 to 3 gms. of the pomegranate rind's powder and swallow this powder with water. In a few hours you will feel the desired relief.

VENERAL DISEASES

Kharbooza or water-melon offers good treatment for these sort of diseases in which the heat of the body increases tremendously because of the infection. The juice of Tarbooz is a good diuretic and through urine body heat is lessened in the body by taking it out of the body. Since all these diseases damage the body by creating heat, Tarbooz (Water Melon) juice is a good remedy. The more the patient urinates, the earlier he should be cured. Alternatively add the cucumber juice in Kalami Shora (salt petre) and make the patient drink it twice a day for quick relief, But one should avoid having fried things, liquor, etc.

WEAKNESS IN GENERAL

For general tonic, Cheeku is the ideal fruit. Have about 6 or 8 Cheekus a day. Still better, if you have these Cheekus after breakfast and lunch and apple juice in the afternoon. Cheeku would provide the necessary strength and apple juice would fill the body up by flesh. But make sure that neither the cheekus nor the apples should be raw or overripe. In just a week's time your body would become powerful and glowing with pink health. But during the period you must tire yourself physically so that these juices provide the necessary fillip to the body.

WHOPPING COUGH

Grate off the small bristles normally found on the stone of kalami mangoes. About a handful would be sufficient. Now burn these bristles to ashes form. When cool, preserve it in a bottle. Now, daily in the night take two gms. of this ash by mixing it with honey and give it to the patient for licking it after adding just a drop of garlic juice. This is tried and tested combination to clear the throat and chest congestion and cure this disease, which normally afflicts children.

WORMS IN INTESTINES

For getting rid of these worms, no need to eat fruits but their rinds. Although it might sound rather unusual, yet it is a tested remedy. Collect the rinds of pomegranates and oranges. Dry them and grind them. Now take just two or three grammes of this rind powder, mix it in about 50 gms. of separated whey or chhach and add salt according to taste. Adding salt is essential as salt kills these worms easily. Have this dose twice or thrice a day. In a couple of days you would be cured of this disease. Having shahtoot (camelemy) is also beneficial.

WOUNDS IN INTESTINES

Those who do not fully munch their food and have hard things in the meals, that too at irregular hours, suffer from this problem. To heal up the wounds in intestines, quince or quince seeds are ideal to heal up these wounds. Just eat a spoonful of these grains and allow them to get dissolved in your mouth. The saliva would be quite thick like gum. You must continue to suck these grain and in a couple of days these wounds of intestines would heal up. But during this period take no solid food.

WEAK EYE-SIGHT

Extract the juice of two small and juicy, sweet oranges, add a little of black pepper powder and drink the juice in the afternoon, preferably about two hours after your lunch. But one or two doses would not give the desired relief. Continue the treatment for about one and a half month days to get back your powerful eye-sight.

■

25

Water in Early Morning— A Tonic for All

Water is panacea for chronic and incurable diseases. Rise early from bed. Do not wash your face and mouth as you do normally. Sit comfortably and drink four large glasses of water. Do not take any thing for 45 minutes. You can wash your face and brush your mouth after drinking water.

Always drink water after an hour of breakfast and meals. Regular intake of water in early morning gives relief in following diseases:

1. Diabetes
2. Acne, Boils
3. Headache
4. Blood pressure
5. Old age and wrinkles
6. Arthritis
7. Paralysis problem of ladies
8. Anaemia
9. Heart diseases, Faintness
10. Cold, Cough, Asthma, Bronchitis
11. Obesity
12. Meningitis
13. Disorders of liver
14. Tuberculosis
15. Disorders of the eye
16. Irregular menstruation
17. Urinary problems, Stones, etc.
18. Hyperacidity Asthma, Bronchitis
19. Gastric trouble and diseases concerned with back, Spine
20. Cancer of ovary
21. Swelling, Fever

22. Digestive disorders

23. Piles

24. Diseases caused by Vata, Pitta, Cough.

25. Mental weakness, etc.

If sick persons or soft natured persons with a delicate physique are unable to take four glasses of water at a stretch, they should start from one or two glasses and then gradually they should start taking four glasses. Take four glasses of water regularly. Experiments have proved that different diseases can be cured within the time given below by its regular use:

Hypertension	-	Within one month
Gastric trouble	-	Within ten days
Cancer	-	Within six months
Constipation	-	Within ten days
Diabetes	-	Within one month
TB	-	Within three months
Leucorrhoea	-	Within one month
Paralysis	-	Within three months

Other diseases described above may be cured within four to six months according to their nature. Drinking four glasses of water does not have any ill-effects on health. Only urge to pass urine will be great and you will pass urine in large quantities frequently. Passing of stool will be easy and complete. It will facilitate the expulsion of the accumulated waste matter very effectively and leave you fresh. Besides hydrotherapy certain other measures or house hold remedies are also advised for such disorders.

Some Important Facts

1. Never drink water before passing urine or just after passing urine.

2. Passing urine after meals prevents formation of stones.

3. Stand on forefoot and then pass urine. This posture prevents formation of stones.

4. Water contained in copper vessel is hundred times more useful.

5. Take juice of one lemon in a glass of warm water before going to bed. It gives relief in Coryza.

6. Take juice of one lemon and tea spoon of honey in warm water in morning. It helps in curing obesity and improves complexion.

7. In early morning, chew five leaves of Neem (Azadiracta indica) and Holy Tulsi (Ocimum basilium) and drink a glass of water after chewing these leaves. This can prevent you from carcinoma (Cancer) and plague too.

8. Take a little rice (raw-one or two tea spoons) with a glass of water to cure liver disorders.

9. The water kept in a Shankh for a whole night is remedy for Stammering speech. Continue this for four to six months.

Role of Water on Stomach

There is secretion of stomachic juice in stomach to digest food. The more genuine the stomachic juice, the better digestion of food.

If someone takes liquid whether it is water, wine or beer the stomachic juice will not remain genuine. It would be adulterated by the intake of water, wine or beer and would not be effective in digestion of food.

Similarly, if some person takes water six or eight times while taking his meal, it would liquidate stomachic juice so much that it would not be able to act as digestive juice.

Do not take water at all during meals. If you have to take it, take very small quantity of it, so that genuine stomachic juice may be absorbed in all eaten food.

If you feel thirsty after one hour or more of taking food, please take water in limited quantity. Body especially stomach needs water at interval from time to time to liquidate its juice, to increase its quantity and to absorb the solid material (food). The body itself informs whenever it needs it. Sometimes, the desire to take water is slow and sometimes it is very fast. One should be particular about intake whether it is from healthy or sick stomach. One should take it as much as it is sufficient and good for health.

It should be taken at equal intervals of time especially when one is suffering from fever. One should not take a glass of water at a stretch but each five or ten minutes in less quantity. Intake of water at a stretch by a patient of fever, will not quench his thirst, rather it would increase other symptoms of illness.

Water taken in less quantity is at once accepted and absorbed by stomach. Repetition of its intake at each half-an-hour produces juice in more quantity and removes whole dullness and constipation by flowing in body and intestines. It cools them also.

One can use luke-warm water or cold water according to its taste.

Use of Water

1. Saline water is necessary in dehydration caused by cholera, fever, diabetes, diarrhoea, etc.

2. It is useful to take water with salt, sugar, lemon and honey. Patients of kidney diseases should use water with salt in supervision of some naturopath.

3. Some of vegetables, water of pulse, sharbat of lemon and juice etc. contain water. They give us minerals and salts along with water.

■ ■ ■

More titles are available in

HEALTH SERIES

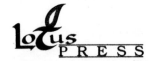

Lotus PRESS

4263, Street No.3, Ansari Road,
Daryaganj, New Delhi-110002
Ph.: 32903912, 23280047, 9811594448
E-mail: lotus_press@sify.com
Website: www.lotuspress.co.in